Compendium
of Clinical Skills for
Student Nurses

Compendium of Clinical Skills for Student Nurses

Edited by

Ian Peate, MA, BEd (Hons), EN(G), RGN, DipN, RNT, LLM

Associate Head of School (Recruitment and Marketing/Professional
Academic Development), School of Nursing and Midwifery,
University of Hertfordshire

W

WHURR PUBLISHERS
LONDON AND PHILADELPHIA

© 2005 Whurr Publishers Ltd

First published 2005
Whurr Publishers Ltd
19b Compton Terrace, London N1 2UN, England and
325 Chestnut Street, Philadelphia PA 19106, USA

British Library Cataloguing in Publication Data

A catalogue record for this book is available from the British
Library.

ISBN 186156 469 4

Printed and bound in the UK by Athenaeum Press Limited,
Gateshead, Tyne & Wear.

Contents

Contributors

David John Briggs, MSC, BA (Hons), DPSN, RGN, NDN (cert), PWT, PGCE (NMC recorded), ILTM, Senior Lecturer, School of Nursing and Midwifery, University of Hertfordshire

Debbie Davies, MSC, BSC, PGCE (FE), RGN, RNT, School of Nursing and Midwifery, University of Hertfordshire

Christine Gault, MSC, RN, RCNT, RNT, PGCE, PCDE, School of Nursing and Midwifery, University of Hertfordshire

Mary Greeno, MA, BSC (Hons), PGCE, RN, SCM, RCNT, RNT, ILTHE, School of Nursing and Midwifery, University of Hertfordshire

Laureen Hemming, BA (Open), BPhil (Complementary Health Care), RGN, RCNT, DipN, PGCEA, Senior Lecturer, School of Nursing and Midwifery, University of Hertfordshire

Jackie Hulse, MSC, BA (Hons), RGN, PGCE, Senior Lecturer, School of Nursing and Midwifery, University of Hertfordshire

Jerry Lancaster, BSC (Chemistry with Microbiology), RGN, Senior Lecturer, School of Nursing and Midwifery, University of Hertfordshire

Janet G. Migliozzi, MSC, BSC (Hons), RGN, PGCE (HE), ILTHE, Senior Lecturer, School of Nursing and Midwifery, University of Hertfordshire

M. Nair, MSC, BSC (Hons), DipN, RNT, certEd, RGN, RMN, ILTHE, Senior Lecturer, School of Nursing and Midwifery, University of Hertfordshire

Ian Peate, MA, BEd (Hons), EN(G), RGN, DipN, RNT, LLM, Associate Head of School (Recruitment and Marketing/Professional Academic Development), School of Nursing and Midwifery, University of Hertfordshire

Lynn Teresa Quinlivan, BSC (Hons), RGN, PGCE, Senior Lecturer, School of Nursing and Midwifery, University of Hertfordshire

Jane Say, MSC, BSC, PGDE, RN, RNT, Senior Lecturer, School of Nursing and Midwifery, University of Hertfordshire

Lynda Elizabeth Sibson, MSC, RGN, RSCN, Asthma Diploma, Nurse Practitioner Diploma, PGCE (HE), Senior Lecturer, School of Nursing and Midwifery, University of Hertfordshire and Independent Nurse Consultant, Hertfordshire

Dedication

This book is dedicated to the memory of Elaine Andrews, Head of Department – Nursing and Adult Health.

Preface

This book has been written for students in order to help them find their way through the many clinical issues that they may face when nursing adults on wards, in clinics and in the community on a daily basis. The text is based on the sole aim of the *Code of Professional Conduct* (Nursing and Midwifery Council [NMC] 2002) – to provide safe and effective care in order to protect the public.

The book encourages students to provide care that is safe and effective and also helps them to assimilate knowledge gained and apply this to the skills needed by the nurse when providing patient care. The information in the book is offered in order to assist the student while on clinical placement and also takes into account the fact that they have academic work to produce for their educational institution, so it is laid out in an easy-to-use format. We do not intend the reader to read the text from cover to cover, but envisage students dipping in and out of it, when clinical issues or concerns emerge.

The text adopts Roper et al.'s (1996) 'activities of living model for nursing' to guide and steer students through the caring and clinical procedures that they perform for and with their patients. Roper et al.'s (1996) model of nursing is used in many clinical areas in the UK, Republic of Ireland, Australia and some European countries; we believe that the framework used is a valuable one for the delivery of care.

Each chapter examines and focuses on an activity of living; however, it must be noted that each activity will impinge on the others, so they are all interrelated. All chapters explore various nursing skills associated with the particular activity of living that the student encounters when in clinical practice. It is anticipated that the information given will encourage students to delve further, to explore the issues discussed and to reflect on their practice.

The chapters also provide the reader with a practical focus, underpinning the theory of nursing – the art and science of caring. Throughout the text the reader is reminded that the nurse is accountable for his or her actions and omissions at all times.

A glossary of the terms used in the text is given in Appendix I; this should assist students to find their way through the intricacies associated with nursing and medical terminology. Appendix II provides 'normal' values to help students appreciate 'abnormal/altered' blood and biochemical results.

The chapters

Chapter 1 sets the scene and provides the reader with insight into the challenges that face nurses in the twenty-first century. The key aim of this chapter is to outline the roles and responsibilities of the nurse with reference to the NMC. Professional nurse regulation, the nursing register and the nurse's duty of care are discussed and clinical examples provided to help the reader understand and appreciate the complexities of professional nursing practice. Chapter 1 addresses important issues surrounding the ethical and legal implications for care delivery, and discusses important concepts such as advocacy, confidentiality and autonomy. Statutory and other government directives are described and the impact that they may have on care delivery is considered. A useful diagrammatic representation of the structure of the NHS is supplied. Chapter 1 concludes by reminding the reader that the best interests of the patient must always come first.

Chapter 2 provides the reader with the building blocks of nursing practice – the nursing process and an introduction to nursing models. Practical examples are given that will help the reader prepare and implement nursing care plans. Chapter 2 explains how the complex activity of assessment is carried out and how to plan care by setting goals that are patient centred and realistic. The act of carrying out care according to a care plan is explained and, finally, the reader is encouraged to provide nursing care that can be measured and evaluated.

Chapter 3 considers safety and draws on current thinking in risk management. Three key/specific areas are highlighted and discussed in detail: drug administration, prevention of falls, infection prevention and control. Methods used to minimize risks related to these three themes are explored. Maintaining a safe environment depends not only on the infrastructure, but also on the equipment and materials used. Chapter 3 points out clearly that all health-care personnel, irrespective of the setting, are responsible for maintaining a safe environment.

Chapter 4 on communication provides much practical advice for those who are new to nursing practice. It is central to all other chapters and suggests that, if the nurse is unable to communicate effectively with his or her patients, the patient is at risk of substandard, if not dangerous, care.

Chapter 5 considers the activity of breathing and starts by guiding the reader through the essential anatomy and physiology of the respiratory system. It draws on the content of other chapters to explain how to communicate with a breathless patient and how to assess the complex activity of breathing. Common respiratory diseases are described and the nursing care needed to help assist the patient outlined. Practical examples for specimen collection and the importance of documenting findings are also discussed.

Eating and drinking are complex activities of living. Two chapters, Chapters 6 and 7, are dedicated to these important fundamental activities. Current thinking about nutrition and nutritional assessment is described in detail, giving the reader a thorough insight into these activities of living, which are responsible for sustaining life. By understanding the complex principles discussed in Chapter 6 the reader should be able to deliver the care required for those patients who have particular care needs, in order to maintain their eating and drinking needs. The roles of the nurse and the multidisciplinary team are described in detail. Chapter 7, in particular, describes the practical elements associated with eating and drinking.

Urinary and faecal elimination are discussed in Chapter 8. An overview of the gastrointestinal and renal tracts is provided in order to explain how eliminatory needs can be met. Several more common diseases are discussed – diseases that the nurse may come across on a regular basis. Chapter 8, as in other chapters, draws on the assessment aspect of nursing and in particular provides the reader with advice about practical nursing interventions. Stoma care and urinary catheterization are described, with hints and tips provided to help the novice nurse begin to manage these aspects of care. Chapter 8 considers the patient in a holistic manner and, as such, deliberates on both the physical and the psychosocial aspects of care.

Chapter 9 details the needs of the patient from a personal cleansing and dressing perspective. It takes the reader through the activity in detail and focuses on the need to help patients maintain their personal hygiene according to their own personal preferences, practices and cultural perspective. The maintenance of hygiene is vitally important for the physical, psychological, emotional and social well-being of the patient. Often this activity is seen as 'basic' care; however, it undermines the significance of the activity and the importance that it has for patients who may be unable to meet their own hygiene needs. Chapter 9 concludes with a plea for this aspect of nursing to receive the recognition it richly deserves because it constitutes essential patient care.

Maintaining body temperature is discussed in Chapter 10, which explains the dynamics associated with thermoregulation and the role that the nurse plays in ensuring that the patient's body temperature is maintained as appropriate. For all forms of life, temperature is a fundamental issue and human beings are no exception to this. Too high a temperature will place the patient in danger, and too low a temperature can be equally detrimental to the patient's well-being. To help the nurse assess the temperature effectively, for appropriate actions to be taken if there is an anomaly in the findings, the various body temperature sites and the various techniques associated with these sites are detailed.

All activities of living are associated with mobility, and Chapter 11 explains this association with movement and mobility, i.e. non-verbal communication in the form of facial expression, breathing and the exchange of gases. It also explains how the musculoskeletal system provides this movement and that mobility is an intrinsic aspect of living. Nurses need to understand the fundamental aspects associated with the musculoskeletal system and how this operates in order to assist and promote the activity of mobility. Chapter 11 outlines how the musculoskeletal system operates. It goes on to explore this activity and provides the nurse with the skills needed to promote effective mobility. Chapter 11 clearly explains the dangers to both nurse and patient if unsafe practice is adopted. Finally, it considers some of the problems frequently associated with patients who are unable to mobilize or move freely.

Chapter 12 begins by asking the reader 'Why does a nurse discuss "occupation", working patterns and leisure interests when admitting or assessing a patient? What are "work and play"? How can they be affected by illness and accident?' It then goes on to explain that such questions are vital if the nurse is to give due consideration to the 'whole' patient. Several key issues are identified and discussed that will help the nurse provide holistic care. A sociological approach is used, and the psychological and social implications that work, leisure and unemployment may have on an individual's quality of life are also included.

In Chapter 13 the issue of sexuality is deliberated. This activity is often neglected by nurses because it has the potential to cause embarrassment and anxiety for both the nurse and the patient. Sex and sexuality are central to what humans are and, as such, nurses are in danger of ignoring a large aspect of the patient's being if they ignore his or her sexuality and any issues surrounding his or her sexual health needs. Chapter 13 provides an insight into this complex activity of living.

Sleeping is discussed in Chapter 14 and it provides the reader with an understanding of the pathophysiology of sleep. Pointers are offered that will enable the nurse to help a patient sleep. This activity of living is often neglected by health-care professionals, and the author raises the important issue of sleep deprivation and the effects that this has on an individual's quality of life.

Finally, Chapter 15 addresses the issue of death and dying. It provides much practical advice to the nurse who may be facing death for the first time. Death and dying can be an upsetting event for all concerned: patient, family and nurse. Chapter 15 considers the care of a person facing death and loss, and the psychological, physical, spiritual and religious needs, and social support are also addressed. There is a discussion about religious and cultural needs after death. After reading Chapter 15, the nurse should gain more insight into this often taboo subject in order to offer closer, more effective support to the patient and those closest to him or her.

It is hoped that this text will whet the appetite and, in so doing, will encourage the reader to delve further into the rewarding and privileged profession of nursing.

References

Nursing and Midwifery Council (2002) Code of Professional Conduct. London: NMC.
Roper, N., Logan, W.W. and Tierney, A.J. (1996) The Elements of Nursing: A model for nursing based on a model of living, 4th edn. Edinburgh: Churchill Livingstone.

Acknowledgements

My grateful appreciation goes to many fine people. I would like to express my specific gratitude to my brother Anthony Peate, who contributed to many of the illustrations, and to Jussi Lahtinen and Frances Cohen.

CHAPTER 1

Contemporary nursing

LYNN TERESA QUINLIVAN

In today's society the central role of a nurse is to deliver high-quality, appropriate care to patients, within a variety of care settings. The role of the nurse is dynamic, continually evolving, in all aspects of health care.

Nursing is associated with caring and helping, and the role of the nurse is often to help the patient achieve or carry out those activities of living that they are unable to do for themselves. Attempting to define nursing is very difficult because there are many facets associated with the role and function of the nurse. There is one particular definition of nursing that has been used since the 1960s – the definition provided by Henderson (1966):

> The unique function of the nurse is to assist the individual, sick or well, in performance of those activities contributing to health or its recovery (or to a peaceful death) that he would perform unaided if he had the necessary strength, will or knowledge and to do this in such a way as to help him gain independence as rapidly as possible.

Henderson's definition is concise and to the point; it appears to encompass many of the roles that the nurse performs, e.g. carer and health educator. This definition could be seen as the nature of nursing.

In this chapter several interlinking sections give the reader an insight into the challenges that face nurses in the twenty-first century.

The role of the nurse and professional accountability

In this section there is a brief discussion relating to the various roles the nurse undertakes. Five distinct areas emerge:

(1) accountability
(2) professionalism
(3) government influences
(4) patients
(5) employers.

The Nursing and Midwifery Council

The Nursing and Midwifery Council (NMC) has taken over the responsibility for the professional regulation of nurses, midwives and health visitors from the UK Central Council (UKCC) and the associated four national boards, which were established in 1979 but have now been superseded.

The NMC has five key functions, four of which were identified under the UKCC. The first key function is the establishment of rules and defined learning outcomes for pre-registration nurse training programmes and the establishment of standardized guidance for 'post-registration education and practice' (PREP). These standards stipulate that all registered practitioners who wish to remain active on the NMC Register must have undertaken a minimum of 35 hours of continuing professional development over a 3-year time period (UKCC 2000).

The second key function is the continuing development of nurses', midwives' and health visitors' appreciation of their professional roles and responsibilities, and the opportunities for professional recognition. These objectives are clearly stated in the *Code of Professional Conduct* (NMC 2002), which states:

> As a registered nurse, midwife or health visitor, you are personally accountable for your practice. In caring for patients and clients you must:
>
> * Respect the patient or client as an individual
> * Obtain consent before you give any treatment or care
> * Protect confidential information
> * Co-operate with others in the team
> * Maintain your professional knowledge and competency
> * Be trustworthy
> * Act to identify and minimise risk to patients and clients.

The third key function relates to professional conduct. The NMC, similarly to its predecessor, the UKCC, seeks to protect society from individuals who are not capable of delivering appropriate safe nursing care to patients and clients. Beverley Allitt is an extreme example of a nurse who was not fit to practise. Beverley Allitt was an enrolled nurse convicted in 1994 of the murder of four of her child patients, and the attempted murder of three others. She failed in her duty of care to her clients and her actions had severe implications for public confidence, accountability and trust in the nursing profession.

The fourth objective is to ensure that the UKCC is a cost-effective, efficient and financially viable organization.

The creation of the NMC has led to the development of a fifth key function. This relates to quality assurance, standard setting and monitoring of educational programmes, which lead to the achievement of a 'registerable or recordable qualification' (NMC 2002). This overarching objective has seen the development of partnerships between 'educational purchasers', such as the workforce development confederations, quality assurance organizations and the quality assurance agency. Institutions for higher education (e.g. universities) are also actively involved, as are the service providers from the independent sector and NHS sector. Finally, other professional regulatory bodies are also involved within the framework, e.g. the General Medical Council. Consequently validation, monitoring and review of nurse education are easily identifiable as a core function of the NMC.

The NMC Register

All nurses, midwives and specialist community public health nurses who wish to practise in the UK must be on the NMC Register; this is a legal requirement. The key purpose for the professional register is to ensure that the NMC is carrying out its role of public protection. The public can be confident that the registered nurses and midwives who care for them are properly qualified and fit for practice (Thewlis 2004).

Alterations to the professional register have taken place as a result of the Nursing and Midwifery Order (2001). The new register will have three parts to it, where previously there were 15:

1. Nurses
2. Midwives
3. Community public health nurses.

The government

In addition to their responsibilities to the regulatory body of the NMC, nurses are accountable to the 'stakeholders', i.e. the general public and the government, for providing effective, efficient, high-quality care.

Since the inception of the NHS in 1948, much debate has surrounded government funding and target setting. Government targets such as reductions in waiting lists, and additional financial resources for certain services such as a winter bed crisis, engender and inflame political opinion and debate about the cost-effectiveness and quality of patient provisions. Present-day government initiatives to involve the public in the development of a health-care service for the twenty-first century are discussed later.

The general public

Nurses are accountable for the delivery of appropriate care to their patients in a variety of care settings, i.e. institutional settings, such as hospitals, and community settings, such as day-care facilities. The level of expertise at which an individual delivers this care will vary, depending on the training/education that the nurse has received.

In the *Code of Professional Conduct* (NMC 2002) the registered practitioners' delegation of responsibility to unqualified staff, and the accountability of that registered practitioner, are stated thus:

You may be expected to delegate care delivery to others who are not registered nurses or midwives. Such delegation must not compromise existing care but must be directed to meeting the needs and serving the interests of patients and clients. You remain accountable for the appropriateness of the delegation, for ensuring that the person who does the work is able to do it and that adequate supervision or support is provided.

Consequently, those involved in patient care should only undertake tasks for which they have received appropriate training/education. In the case of delivering key aspects of nursing care, e.g. washing and feeding a patient, this may be as part of a formal programme of study such as the National Vocational Qualification in Health Care Studies.

The employer

Finally, nurses are accountable to their employer under a contract of employment. Under terms of employment there is an understanding that nurses will act in a responsible manner when they carry out their duties. NHS trusts have their own policies and procedures, which are designed to ensure that patients are protected from harm. The term 'vicarious liability', a very complex concept, refers to situations whereby the employer accepts responsibility for the faults of its employees. However, if the employee is found not to have followed an accepted procedure or protocol, e.g. the trust's drug administration policy, then the trust is not legally liable for the employee's error.

Duty of care and professional nurse regulation

The duty of care owed to the patient by the nurse and continuing professional development are outlined in this section. The *Code of Professional Conduct* (NMC 2002) applies directly to qualified nurse practitioners; however, the principles that it sets out, of good practice and duty of care, apply to all those directly involved in patient care.

Lord Aitkin defined duty of care as follows (*Donoghue v Stevenson* 1932):

> You must take reasonable care to avoid acts or omissions which you can reasonably foresee would be likely to injure your neighbour.

The definition of what is reasonable originates from the Bolam test, where the case of *Bolam v Friern Hospital Management Committee* 1957 resulted in the following legal ruling:

> The test is the standard of the ordinary skilled man exercising and professing to have that special skill. A man need not possess the highest expert skill at the risk of being found negligent . . . . It is sufficient if he exercises the skill of an ordinary competent man exercising that particular art.

The regulatory process and the regulation of nurses by the NMC are designed to encourage life-long learning through the construction of a portfolio of evidence. Nurses are required to re-register every 3 years, at which time the Council can request to see evidence of continuing professional development. A continuing professional development portfolio may include the following sections.

Evidence of professional learning

The minimum requirement for registered nurses is 35 hours' study within a 3-year period. These study days must include an annual update in relation to moving and handling and cardiopulmonary resuscitation.

In addition to these mandatory study days there is a requirement for practitioners to demonstrate evidence of continuing professional learning by attending study sessions relevant to their areas of clinical practice, e.g. a district nurse may choose to attend a tissue viability study day and then write a short reflective account which enables him or her to consider how this knowledge can be applied within clinical practice.

Life events

This section may include an aspect of family life that has had some impact on an individual's working life, e.g. getting married, changing job, or completion of a period of study that has resulted in new and challenging responsibilities.

Critical incidents and personal reflection

Critical incidents are incidents that the nurse has observed and/or taken part in which have affected her or him, e.g. looking after a patient who subsequently dies. The positive aspects of learning are not always apparent at the time; however, by using a framework such as Gibbs' reflective cycle (Gibbs 1988) (see Chapter 4 for more discussion of Gibbs' cycle) an individual can look retrospectively at the incident and analyse subsequent learning.

The regulation of nursing practice by the NMC also relates to individual practitioners whose actions or clinical competencies have been subject to investigation. Often this is termed 'professional misconduct'. When allegations have been made against a practitioner, this is taken seriously by the NMC who will decide whether an investigation into the practitioner's actions or omissions necessitates a misconduct hearing. If the NMC, after the misconduct hearing, deems the action or omissions to be serious enough, it has the ability to remove or suspend the practitioner from the professional register. The overriding aim in taking such serious action is to protect the public.

One other key function of the NMC is to validate programmes of study provided by educational institutions such as universities. The aim is to ensure that the theoretical and practical components of a programme fulfil set criteria for the admission of graduates to the professional register. The NMC representatives (they are known as 'visitors') visit the educational institution and clinical areas to which student nurses are allocated, ensuring that the learning experience is appropriate and meaningful, and that practice assessors and mentors adequately support student nurses within the clinical environment.

Ethical and legal considerations in relation to the delivery of care

In this section common terms that you may meet in practice are defined and related to examples of patient care. Every aspect of nursing practice is associated with some form of ethical action and often this is bound up in law. All citizens are subject to the law:

> You must respect patients' rights and clients' autonomy - their right to decide whether or not to undergo any health care intervention - even where a refusal may result in harm or death to themselves.

> NMC (2002)

Advocacy

Advocacy, according to Mason and Whitehead (2003), is defined as:

> Providing active support for the patient in the health care environment. A central role of the nurse is to act as a go-between, representing the patient when they cannot represent themselves, for the effective operation of the doctor-patient relationship.

An example of advocacy is when a patient has expressed concerns in relation to his or her medical condition, treatment or ongoing care, but does not feel able to express his or her concerns directly to the appropriate member of the multidisciplinary team. The patient asks the nurse to raise their concerns with the relevant member of the team, which could be a doctor, physiotherapist, occupational therapist, dietitian or district nurse.

Autonomy

Mason and Whitehead (2003) consider the key attributes of autonomy to be 'the capacity to think, make decisions and to take action independently of others'. Autonomy can be subdivided into:

- Autonomy of thought: in this case the patient can engage in all aspects of thinking without interference from others.
- Autonomy of will: the patient has the freedom to decide and make choices in respect of medical and/or nursing interventions.

- Autonomy of action: the actions that the patient or client chooses to make are dependent on being in a reasonable and rational state of mind (Mason and Whitehead 2003).

For example, a patient makes the choice to walk to a bathroom for an assisted wash, rather than sitting in a chair by the side of the bed in a ward. The patient may well discuss issues relating to a feeling of greater privacy afforded within a bathroom rather than a curtained area within a ward.

Beneficence

Mason and Whitehead (2003) suggest that beneficence is:

> To show by actions a positive kindness and to behave in a way that produces a positive outcome for the person.

When caring for a patient the nurse ensures that the patient wishes to have the planned intervention, e.g. the delivery of appropriate fundamental care to a patient who is unable to wash him- or herself. The nurse is required to ensure that the planned intervention is in accordance with the patient's wishes, needs and desires, so, if the patient refuses or declines to have a wash, the nurse must respect the client's wishes.

Confidentiality

> Confidentiality refers to respecting other people's secrets. Confidentiality involves the elements of trust, which is required from both parties in both giving honest information and maintaining its secrecy.
>
> Mason and Whitehead (2003)

For example, a patient informs you of their fears in relation to medical treatment. It may be appropriate for you to share the fact that they have a fear with other members of the multidisciplinary team. However, it would not be appropriate for the nurse or health-care assistant to divulge the precise details of any conversation without first gaining the patient's consent. To do so without the patient's consent may be classed as a breach of confidentiality.

Consent

Consent is subdivided into three sections:

1. Valid consent occurs when a patient or client gives consent voluntarily and under no duress, e.g. a patient agrees to a blood test.
2. Written consent, e.g. the patient gives written consent to an operation, or some other investigation not necessarily requiring a general anaesthetic.
3. Implied consent: non-verbal communication, e.g. the patient implies this consent by rolling up a pyjama sleeve to allow the nurse to take the patient's blood pressure.

Dimond (2003) considers consent to be the following:

> Any adult, mentally competent person has the right in law to consent to any touching of his person. If he is touched without consent or other lawful justification, then the person has the right of action in the civil courts of suing for trespass to the person – battery where the person is actually touched, assault where he fears that he will be touched.

Empowerment

Empowerment can be defined as (Macpherson 2004):

> The engagement of individuals in decisions about their health and about the diagnosis, treatment and aftercare.

The individual client has the right to make decisions about his or her treatment; health-care professionals have a duty to ensure that the patient has adequate knowledge and understanding to enable the patient to make an informed judgement, e.g. a patient may refuse to have intravenous fluids, despite an inadequate oral intake; this action may be detrimental to the patient's health. However, if the consequences of not having an adequate oral intake have been explained to the patient in language that he or she understands, the patient is said to be making an informed choice when refusing to have intravenous fluids.

Non-maleficence

'Non-maleficence is to do no harm to others' (Mason and Whitehead 2003), e.g. if a patient declines to sit in a chair, stating that he or she finds it uncomfortable to do so, it would be an inappropriate action for the nurse to then move the patient out of bed into a chair.

Nursing hierarchy

Within a clinical setting it is common to find a nursing hierarchy. The job titles within a typical hierarchy, along with the roles and responsibilities of nurses holding these titles, are described in this section.

Ward managers

The ward manager is responsible for the 24-hour delivery of care to patients within a designated care setting. Consequently, a ward manager will have a wide range of responsibilities, which may vary from the day-to-day management of an off-duty rota to the management of ward budgets. The ward manager may be responsible for the recruitment and selection of new members of staff. Part of the role is also ensuring that all staff members develop and retain appropriate clinical skills, so the ward manager must enable qualified and unqualified staff to attend clinical study days that meet their professional and academic needs. Such developmental objectives may have been highlighted during the yearly appraisal cycle, for which the ward manager is also responsible. The ward manager may also be actively involved in clinical audits and the writing of policies and procedures relating to their field of expertise.

Senior ward sisters/charge nurses

A senior ward sister or charge nurse will usually be a registered general nurse with at least 2 years' experience as a junior sister/charge nurse. A senior ward sister or charge nurse would be expected to hold additional qualifications depending on the speciality within which she or he is working, e.g. a charge nurse in an intensive care setting would be required to hold a qualification relating to intensive care nursing as well as the post-registration certificate for mentoring and assessing student nurses. A senior ward sister or charge nurse will be responsible for the delivery of 24-hour care; this may include staffing arrangements, the implementation of policies and procedures, and the compilation of data for clinical audits which relate to government directives such as *A First Class Service* (Department of Health [DoH] 1998).

Junior ward sisters/charge nurses

A junior sister is a registered nurse with at least 2 years' experience as a senior staff nurse and an appropriate secondary qualification, e.g. a charge nurse working within an orthopaedic setting may hold an additional qualification related to orthopaedic nursing. A junior sister will be expected to undertake the management of a designated clinical environment. In addition, she or he may be involved in the implementation of government directives such as the 'fractured neck of femur pathway' (DoH 2000). A junior sister or charge nurse will be required to supervise and develop the clinical expertise and competencies of junior members of the nursing staff, e.g. newly qualified staff nurses, student nurses or health-care assistants; it is common for a junior sister or charge nurse to hold the Mentorship Preceptorship certificate in areas where student nurses are allocated.

Senior staff nurses

A senior staff nurse will typically be a registered nurse with at least 12 months' experience as a junior staff nurse. Senior staff nurses are responsible for ensuring that safe appropriate care is delivered to patients and their families. In carrying out their duties, senior staff nurses are required to assess, plan, implement and evaluate the care that is provided to patients over a recognized time period, e.g. an early shift. In carrying out their duties, senior staff nurses are expected to take an active role in liaising with other members of the multidisciplinary team such as doctors, physiotherapists, district nurses and general practitioners.

Junior staff nurses, D grade

The title of junior staff nurse relates to a newly qualified staff nurse with current nursing and midwifery registration and previous NHS experience, albeit as a student nurse.

Senior health-care assistants, level 3

Under the National Vocational Qualifications (NVQs), there are two levels of training that individuals may choose to access to develop fundamental skills associated with caring for patients. A senior health-care assistant will have successfully completed the level 3 NVQ in Health Care Studies. The role of a senior health-care assistant is to provide fundamental care to patients under the supervision and direction of a qualified practitioner, and to watch over more junior members of the team.

Junior health-care assistants, level 2

Junior health-care assistants will have completed an NVQ in Health Care Studies at level 2 or be undertaking this qualification. A junior health-care assistant will deliver personal care to clients within a variety of care settings under the supervision of senior team members.

Student nurses

Student nurses will undertake a 3-year programme of study that is 50% theory and 50% practice based. Satisfactory completion of both components will enable the student nurse to register as a qualified nurse practitioner.

There are two potential qualifications that are achievable, although often this will depend on the individual higher educational institution: these are either a degree alternatively known as BSC/BSC (HONS) Nursing (Adult/Child/Mental Health) or BSC (HONS) Nursing (Learning Disabilities) and Diploma in Social Work; or a Diploma of Higher Education in Nursing (Mental Health/Learning Disabilities/Child/Adult). These two programmes are organized in a similar manner in the first year of nursing training; this year is known as the Common Foundation Programme and the final two years are the branch-specific aspects of the programme.

District nurses

A district nurse assesses patients within a community setting; this may be the client's home or a facility such as a care home. A district nurse will plan and implement care, maintain associated records and coordinate the workload of the team of which he or she is a member.

Health visitors

A health visitor works with families with specific health and social needs, and consequently liaises as and when appropriate with other health professionals and agencies such as Social Services. Health visitors run child health clinics, providing advice and health education to parents of babies and young children. The health visitor also works with older people, i.e. those aged 65 years and over.

Specialist nurses

Specialist nurses will have a deep understanding of a particular branch of nursing care, e.g. the palliative care nurse possesses deep knowledge in relation to the care, management and symptom control of patients with a terminal illness.

Government directives and organizations

In this section some government directives and organizations are described. The government lays down statutes in law, which relate directly to clinical practice.

Patients' Charter (DoH 1995)

This was introduced to inform the general public of the choices that they have in relation to health care. The Charter (DoH 1995) measures activity within hospitals, e.g. the length of time patients wait to see a consultant in an out-patient department (Komaromy 2001).

Clinical governance

Each individual NHS trust's board of governors is responsible for ensuring that safe and acceptable standards of care are delivered in all areas of clinical and non-clinical practice:

> A framework through which NHS organisations are accountable for continuously improving the quality of their services.
>
> DoH (1998)

Data Protection Act 1998

This Act sets out eight principles which apply to the keeping of computerized data. Employers are responsible for ensuring that data collection systems comply with the provisions as set out within the Act.

As a nurse collecting patient information, it may be appropriate for you to share data with other members of the multidisciplinary team, e.g. if a patient has a drug allergy, the patient has given implied consent when disclosing such information. However, if subsequently research was undertaken in relation to drug allergies, the patient's consent to be involved in the trial cannot be assumed, because the data relate to an in-patient admission not a drug trial.

These principles are designed to ensure that personal data shall be accurate, relevant, held only for specific defined purposes for which the user has been registered, not kept for longer than necessary, and not disclosed to unauthorised persons.

Dimond (2003)

Our Healthier Nation (DoH 1999)

This is an action plan to tackle poor health, in which the government sets out its aims to:

Improve the health of everyone and the health of the worst off in particular.

In *Our Healthier Nation* (DoH 1999) the government puts forward the following four targets to be achieved by 2010:

1. A reduction in the death rates of those under 75 years of age from cancer, by at least a fifth.
2. A reduction in the death rates associated with coronary heart disease and stroke, in those under 75 years of age, by at least two-fifths.
3. A reduction in accidents and serious injury by a tenth.
4. A reduction in the death rates associated with suicide by at least a fifth in line with overarching objectives relating to the treatment of mental illness.

The government explains how it intends to achieve these objectives, principally by increasing funding and encouraging the development of local health initiatives:

A new balance in which people, communities and government work together in partnership to improve health.

DoH (1999)

National Institute for Clinical Excellence (NICE)

One of the functions of this organization, set up in 1999, is to disseminate good clinical practice throughout the NHS, and offer guidelines in relation to research-based practice.

Guidance for clinicians does not override their professional responsibility to make the appropriate decisions in the circumstances of the individual patient.

Dimond (2003)

Commission for Health Improvement

The function of this regulatory body was, first, to provide advice or information, conduct reviews and make reports on arrangements by primary health-care trusts or NHS trusts for the purposes of monitoring and improving the quality of health care for which they are responsible, and, second, to carry out investigations and conduct reviews in relation to the management, provision or quality of, or access to or availability of, particular types of health care for which NHS bodies or service providers have responsibility (Dimond 2003).

The Commission for Health Improvement's function has now been taken over by the Health Care Commission.

The National Health Service Plan (DoH 2000)

The NHS Plan sets out specific targets for NHS trusts to achieve within documented time frames, e.g. the 'fractured neck of femur pathway', which is an integrated care pathway that aims to manage effectively and efficiently the patient's progression from accident and emergency to discharge. Within the provision of this 'fast-track care' is the involvement of members of the multidisciplinary team, such as physiotherapists, occupational therapists, social workers, doctors, nurses, district nurses and hospital-at-home services. The ultimate aim is for those patients to have a shorter in-patient time and an improved community support network upon discharge (Komaromy 2001).

Agenda for Change

The underpinning principles of *Agenda for Change* are the harmonization of terms and conditions for all NHS employees. *Agenda for Change* aims to address the issue of equal pay for work of equal value. It will also mean an end to clinical grading (Royal College of Nursing 2004).

Health Care Commission

The Health Care Commission's remit is to review the quality of care that is currently provided across the NHS and the independent sector, with the aim of ensuring that the care provided meets the prescribed recognized standards, e.g. benchmark statements, standards of clinical excellence as set out by NICE (Health Act 1999). The Health Care Commission will inform patients, the general public, health service employees and health professionals about changes and improvements to local health-care provision (Health Care Commission 2004).

National Health Service Live

This is a programme designed to improve the quality of health care through local projects. These projects are tailor-made and involve joint collaboration between sponsor partners and primary care trusts. One example is the 'virtual healthy living centre', which has been set up in Basildon; its aim is to enable patients to manage their illness within their home environment by utilizing innovative information technology (Donaldson 2004).

The structure of the NHS in England

This section outlines the structure of the NHS in 2004 (Figure 1.1).

Department of Health

The Department of Health supports the government in its plans to reform and provide an integrated and comprehensive range of services based on clinical need, not the ability to pay.

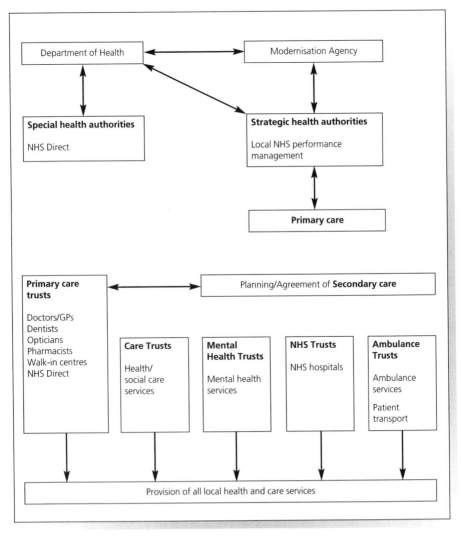

Figure 1.1
The NHS in England. (From
Department of Health 2004.)

Modernisation Agency

Established in 2001, the Agency's remit is to develop 'patient-centred service that gives power to its staff and patients at all levels' (Modernisation Agency 2004). This agency has two core functions: first, to ensure that the NHS meets the needs of its patients in the twenty-first century; second, the Agency is expected to modernize services in an appropriate and meaningful manner, so that the services that the general public requires are those that are accessible and available. The Modernisation Agency is expected to achieve this objective by the integration of services and the development of best practice throughout the NHS, e.g. by clinical governance support teams which will work alongside the primary care development team.

Special health authorities

The National Blood Authority and NHS Direct fall into this category; their remit is the provision of a national service; e.g. NHS Direct provides information, advice and support for patients who are able to access this service via a free telephone number 24 hours a day, 7 days a week (DoH 2004).

Strategic health authorities

In 2002, the government created 28 strategic health authorities. Their function at the present time is to manage local national health services; the strategic health authorities achieve this by developing local improvement plans and ensuring that national priorities such as the development of an integrated stroke care pathway are actively supported (DoH 2001).

Primary care trusts

Primary care trusts manage local health-care services within primary care groups: general practitioners, dentists, opticians and pharmacists. The function of the primary care trusts is thus to ensure that there is adequate provision of services for the general population; this could be NHS hospital services and in-patient and out-patient provisions, or the NHS walk-in centres and mental health services (Commission for Health Improvement 2003).

Mental health trusts

These provide a range of psychological therapies such as bereavement counselling, general health screening within the local community, and in-patient health-care provision for clients, which can, for example, include patients with psychotic illnesses (Commission for Health Improvement 2003).

NHS trusts

Acute trusts

Acute trusts manage hospitals and formulate strategies for the improvement of hospital services; they are also the employers of hospital staff such as doctors, nurses, midwives, health visitors and allied health professionals, e.g. physiotherapists and radiographers (DoH 2004).

Foundation trusts

Foundation trusts are NHS hospitals that have been given a degree of financial and operational independence. The trusts remain within the overarching umbrella of the NHS. However, they are run by members of the public, staff and locally based managers who are able to tailor the services provided to the needs of the local population (DoH 2004).

Ambulance trusts

There are 33 ambulance services covering England, providing access to emergency health care for the general population. The ambulance service operates on three levels, ranging from immediate life-threatening cases to non-emergency responses. Under government strategic plans, certain criteria are set that relate to response times.

Conclusion

In this chapter a generalized overview of nurses' roles and responsibilities in the twenty-first century has been discussed. The nurse's role is complex and embraces the notions of autonomy and accountability. The role of the Nursing and Midwifery Council in relation to the regulation of pre- and post-registration nurse education has been explained, as have nurses' fourfold responsibilities: first to the general public, then their professional organization (NMC), the government and finally their employer.

Nursing has advanced in a variety of ways. The patient, however, must always be at the heart of these advances – first and foremost, the nurse must strive to provide care that is of the highest standard. Professional conduct and performance must also be taken into account (Slevin 2003).

The importance of life-long learning and reflective practice has been introduced, and the causes and consequences of changing government directives in relation to patients' choices have been briefly discussed. Ethical and legal terminology relating to fundamental care has been explained with practical clinical examples. The chapter concluded with a synopsis of the current structure of the NHS and the responsibilities of specific NHS trusts.

Table of cases

Bolam v Friern Hospital Management Committee [1957] 2 All ER 118
Donoghue v Stevenson [1932] AC 562 (HL)

References

Commission for Health Improvement (2003) NHS Performance Ratings: Primary care trusts, mental health trusts, learning disability trusts: 2002/2004. London: Commission for Health Improvement.

Department of Health (1995) The Patients' Charter and You. London: Department of Health.

Department of Health (1998) A First Class Service: Quality in the new NHS. London: Department of Health.

Department of Health (1999) Saving Lives: Our healthier nation. London: Department of Health.

Department of Health (2000) The NHS Plan: A plan for investment. A plan for reform. London: Department of Health.

Department of Health (2001) Shifting the Balance of Power Within the NHS: Securing delivery. London: Department of Health.

Department of Health (2004) The Structure of the NHS (NHS Gateway). London: Department of Health.

Dimond, B. (2003) Legal Aspects of Nursing, 3rd edn. London: Pearson Education.

Donaldson, L. (2004) NHS Live Goes Live (2004/0251). London: Department of Health.

Gibbs G. (1988) Learning by Doing: A guide to teaching and learning methods. Oxford: Further Education Unit, Oxford Polytechnic.

Health Care Commission (Commission for Health Care Audit and Inspection) (2004) Newsletter – July. London: Department of Health.

Henderson, V. (1966) The Nature of Nursing: A definition and its implications for practice, research and education. New York: Macmillan.

Komaromy, C. (ed.) (2001) Dilemmas in UK Health Care. Milton Keynes: Open University Press.

Macpherson, G. (2004) Black's Medical Dictionary. London: A & C Black.

Mason, T. and Whitehead, E. (2003) Thinking Nursing. Milton Keynes: Open University Press.

Modernisation Agency (2004) New Ways of Working: Investing in staff is investing in care. London: The Modernisation Agency.

Nursing and Midwifery Council (2002) Code of Professional Conduct. London: NMC.

Nursing and Midwifery Order (2001) Statutory Instrument Number 253.

Royal College of Nursing (2004) Agenda for Change: Getting prepared. London: Royal College of Nursing.

Slevin, O. (2003) Nursing as a profession. In: Basford, L. and Slevin, O. (eds), Theory and Practice of Nursing: An integrated approach to caring and practice, 2nd edn. London: Nelson Thornes, pp. 97–111.

Thewlis, S. (2004) The new register opens. NMC News 8: 10–11.

United Kingdom Central Council (2000) UKCC and PREP. London: UKCC.

Some helpful websites

Carlisle and District NHS Primary Care Trust (2003) Your Guide to Local Services: www.carlislepct.nhs

Dacorum NHS, Primary Care Trust: www.dacorum-pct.nhs.uk/foi/bodies

Hertfordshire Partnership NHS Trust, Freedom of Information Publication Scheme:

Classes of Information, Class 1: The NHS and how we fit: www.hpt.mhs.uk/foi/classes/1nhs/Default.htm

NHS in England, National Service Frameworks (NSFs): www.nhs.uk/england/aboutTheNHS/nsf/default.cmsx

Nursing and Midwifery Council: www.nmc-uk.org

Royal College of Nursing: www.rcn.org.uk

CHAPTER 2

The nursing process

LYNDA ELIZABETH SIBSON

This chapter centres on the nursing process from a broad perspective, focusing on some of the key concepts that support and inform the nursing process in today's nursing practice. It does not include a detailed discussion about some of the conceptual models of care, but rather looks at some of the key components that underpin the nursing process. It provides a background to the organization of nursing care, with specific reference to Florence Nightingale, who is considered by many to be the founder of nursing. The chapter also includes information related to:

- the organization of nursing care
- the assessment, planning, implementation and evaluation of care
- measurement, observation and communications
- documentation
- nursing care plans.

This chapter aims to dispel some of the myths and confusion surrounding the nursing process, providing readers with a clear overview of this fundamental concept in nursing. Throughout this chapter the term 'individual' will be used instead of patient. This is to reflect that not everyone for whom nurses care is necessarily ill (e.g. people in the community and primary care), but they do need some form of nursing intervention, perhaps as a preventive measure.

Organization of nursing care

Crucial to the delivery of quality individualized nursing care is a method of organizing care, such as the nursing process (Kemp and Richardson 1994). The nursing process was introduced into the UK in 1980. It was initially regarded with some scepticism, partly as a result of its adoption from America, where it had been implemented some years earlier. However, it has now been fully accepted into UK nursing practice and is present, in one form or another, in most clinical areas.

Although the concept of the nursing process has been the cornerstone of professional nursing practice for a number of years, it has been open to misinterpretation, causing confusion among students and novices of nursing practice. However, it is generally recognized as describing a systematic approach to nursing, which comprises a series of steps or stages that refer to the assessment, planning, implementation and evaluation of nursing care (Roper et al. 1993). In this sense, the nursing process is essentially what nurses do when providing individual nursing care. In other words, the nursing process is a *thinking* and *doing* approach that nurses use in their work (Wilkinson 1996).

Nursing in itself is a unique blend of art and science applied to our professional practice as nurses. Nursing was initially task oriented – often a list of tasks to be carried out. This approach was favoured in practice for many years, because nurses were considered to be the 'doctor's handmaiden' – overseen by formidable matrons in large frilly hats and starched aprons! As nurses have emerged as professionals in their own right, the 'science of nursing' has taken precedence, with nursing theory and knowledge seen as essential to achieving a scientific knowledge base in nursing practice (Chinn and Kramer 1995).

Nursing practice in the UK has developed rapidly over the last 30 years. The changes to nurse education, from a hospital to a university setting, and nurses undertaking diplomas and degrees are examples of the development in professionalism. Nursing is currently organized into four specialisms or 'branches'. During the first year of a course, nurses are introduced to all of these specialisms as part of the Common Foundation Programme. The second and third years focus on the branch of choice, which can be adult, children's, or mental health or learning disability nursing. Midwifery and health visiting are regarded as separate professions although still within the nursing family.

With the additional development of nurse practitioners and nurse consultants, this is a long way from our more humble beginnings – or is it?

Florence Nightingale, considered the founder of nursing and the first nursing theorist, based her theories on her own experiences during the Crimean War. During Nightingale's era of the late nineteenth century, unsanitary conditions posed a great health hazard and she concluded that external influences and conditions can prevent, suppress or contribute to death and disease. This was revolutionary at the time, because nurses were not then employed to *think*, just to *do*. Although now highly regarded and respected, during her career her important observations, which she published widely, were ignored by the government of the time (McDonald 2002).

Florence commenced her nursing training at age 31, much to her parents' disquiet, because at the time a career in nursing was associated with working-class women and Florence was from a wealthy and privileged background. After qualifying, she was appointed resident lady superintendent of a hospital for invalid women in Harley Street, London.

With the commencement of the Crimean War in 1853, British soldiers sent into battle were contracting cholera and malaria. Within weeks an estimated 8000 men were suffering from these diseases. Florence, among others, offered her services to help with the epidemic. Her offer was initially rejected, but when a national newspaper (alerted by Florence) publicized the huge cholera death rate among the soldiers there was a public outcry, and the government was forced to change its mind. Florence again volunteered her services and, with 38 colleagues, she was appalled at the conditions that they faced. Injured soldiers were kept in rooms without blankets or decent food. Unwashed, they were still wearing their army uniforms. In these conditions, it was perhaps not surprising that, in army hospitals, war wounds only accounted for one death in six. Diseases such as typhus, cholera and dysentery were the main reasons why the death rate was so high among wounded soldiers.

Against strong military objection for Florence to radically reform these field hospitals, she was again forced to use the British media to highlight the appalling conditions of these wounded soldiers and, after a great deal of publicity, Florence was given the task of organizing the nursing care, and by improving the quality of the sanitation she was able to dramatically reduce the death rate of the soldiers.

After the war, Florence returned to England as a national heroine. She had been deeply moved by the lack of basic hygiene and elementary care that the men received in the British Army and she decided to begin a campaign to improve the quality of nursing in military hospitals.

She published widely on her findings and with the support of friends raised money to improve the quality of nursing, founding the Nightingale School and Home for Nurses at St Thomas' Hospital. She also became involved in the training of nurses for employment in the workhouses which had been established as a result of the 1834 Poor Law Amendment Act. Before her death in 1910, at the age of 90, Florence championed women's rights and campaigned ardently for women to have careers (Nightingale 1969).

The reason that Florence's work was so important was that she used her own form of nursing process to improve the quality of care for the soldiers. Her basic theory was that there was a link between health and the environment, which at the time had not been considered.

She suggested that there were five elements essential for restoring health. These were simply:

(1) pure air
(2) pure water
(3) light

(4) cleanliness
(5) efficient drainage.

She concluded that the *environment* in which her patients were nursed had an impact on their health and she suggested the following factors:

- Physical environment: where the individual is treated
  - ventilation, warmth, cleanliness, light, noise and drainage.
- Psychological environment:
  - affected by a negative physical environment causing stress
  - communication - should be therapeutic, soothing and unhurried.
- Social environment:
  - collecting data about illness and disease prevention
  - components in the physical environment, e.g. clean air, water and drainage.

So, perhaps Florence led the way? She was certainly visionary in collecting data about her patients, planning, implementing and evaluating their care. She even shared this information with other nurses through her books and letters.

Present nursing leaders include a Chief Nursing Officer (CNO) employed by the Department of Health. Nursing's professional bodies include the Royal College of Nursing (RCN), essentially a nursing union, which represents the interests of nurses and nursing. The RCN also provides an educational role and lobbies government on policies to raise the profile of nursing in the UK.

The Nursing and Midwifery Council (NMC) is an organization set up by Parliament to protect the public by ensuring that nurses, midwives and health visitors provide high standards of care to their clients. The NMC maintains a register of qualified nurses, midwives and health visitors. It sets standards for education, practice and conduct, provides advice for nurses, midwives and health visitors, and considers allegations of misconduct or unfitness to practise as a result of ill health. The NMC produces a number of practice guidelines, which are listed at the end of the chapter.

What is the nursing process?

When dealing with a new concept, definitions are always a useful starting point. So the term 'nursing process' is worth separating into its two components: 'nursing' and 'process'. The organization and background to 'nursing' have been described earlier.

A 'process' can be defined as a procedure, method or course of action. It is often used to describe a series of interrelated events that result in an outcome of one kind or another. A process can be applied to practically any aspect of life. The process by which we use a cashpoint machine to remove money from our bank accounts is one example. We have a plastic card, with personalized information stored on it, which we insert into a machine. By entering a four-digit assigned number (called a PIN number) and then selecting a number of options, we can withdraw cash, check our bank balance or perhaps order a bank statement. A sequence of events (possession of a card, a PIN number and a computerized machine) has occurred that results in an outcome.

The nursing process works in similar ways. However, a number of words are used in conjunction with the nursing process that are worth explaining briefly to avoid confusion. These are theory, models, concepts and conceptual models.

Theory

A theory provides a way of looking at a discipline, such as nursing, in clear and explicit terms that can be communicated to others. Therefore, nursing theories help to explain the unique place of nursing within the health-care profession, e.g. how nursing differs from the role of a doctor or physiotherapist.

Models

The word 'model' refers to a system that is not necessarily written in 'tablets of stone', but is flexible, varies over time and should reflect current practice and research. A model should be:

- systematic, e.g. have clear basic systems in place
- based on evidence, e.g. include the latest research findings, current thinking and have an evidence base
- related to concepts
- related to theories and values, e.g. include the relevant theory and accepted professional values (this includes acting professionally, respecting an individual and confidentiality).

Concepts

A 'concept' refers to a formal view or image of something.

Conceptual models

Conceptual models for nursing are therefore formal presentations of some nurses' private views or images of nursing. Conceptual models should:

- identify essential components of the discipline (in this case, nursing)
- show relationships between concepts or other views
- introduce already established theories from other disciplines (such as psychology and sociology).

There are a number of conceptual models that demonstrate the nursing process; examples include:

- Orem's model of self-care (Orem 1980)
- Roy's adaptation model (Roy 1984)
- Neuman's health-care system model (Neuman 1982)
- Peplau's interpersonal model (Peplau 1988)
- Roper's activities of living (ALs) model (Roper et al. 1993).

Putting all these components together, we have the 'nursing process'. As outlined earlier, this chapter focuses on the key components that make up the nursing process rather than looking at individual conceptual models. There are essentially four steps to the nursing process (whichever conceptual model is adopted) and these are now looked at in detail.

Assessment, planning, implementation and evaluation of care

It is worth remembering that all the stages in the nursing process are continuous and interlink with each other, as Figure 2.1 demonstrates. For example, although assessment is the first stage, the individual should be assessed continuously throughout the episode of care – whether in a hospital or in a community setting.

Figure 2.1
The nursing process.

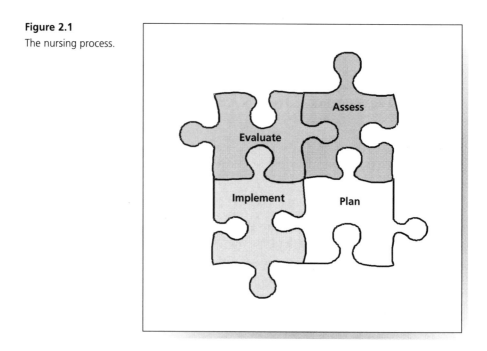

The sample care plan in Table 2.1 provides a simple overview of the information that is required to assess, plan, implement and evaluate care (Roper et al.'s ALs have been used here) and each stage is described below in more detail. A practical example is also used to demonstrate the stages involved in the nursing process. Remember that these are generic and can apply to any conceptual model that is adopted in the particular area of health care in which you find yourself working.

Assessment: what is the problem and what needs to be done?

The first stage in the nursing process is to collect, organize and examine the information about an individual. This information can be collected in a number of ways, using a number of methods. The aim of this stage is to

Table 2.1 Sample care plan

Assess	Plan	Implement	Evaluate
When assessing an individual's needs, the following factors should be taken into consideration:	When writing goals, some factors to remember are:	This part of a care plan needs to show all the nursing interventions. Points to remember are:	This aspect of a care plan is ongoing until a problem has been resolved. Some important facts to remember:
• List individual problems in order of priority • Number each problem • Date each problem • Assess each problem in association with, for example, Roper et al's activities of living	• They must be written in terms of individual achievement, e.g. 'Mr X will state that he feels less anxious' • Write at least one short-term goal • Make each goal measurable, e.g. 'Mr X will show lessened pain with the use of a pain chart' • Each goal should state a target date and time for evaluation	• List specific actions in relation to working towards the set goals • In most cases several actions are required to achieve just one goal • It is often a good idea to cite rationale for actions	• State clearly the time and date of evaluation • Use any measures that were mentioned in aims, e.g. 'Mr X states that his pain is now reduced from 7 to 2 on the pain scale' • For long-term goals explain how much nearer to achieving that goal an individual is • Consider any changes or additions to nursing actions that might have come about

identify clearly the individual's problem(s) so that care can be planned. This information is usually recorded in a care plan. The care plan takes many different formats and varies from hospital to hospital, but it is usually a paper form (although computer-based forms are becoming increasingly popular) which contains basic information.

The collection of this information will often take the form of an interview. Although this is informal, it is an essential part of the nursing process and should be conducted in an area that respects the individual's confidentiality – so as far as possible not within direct earshot of a room full of other people! In a busy hospital ward, this can be difficult, but, by at least pulling the curtains around the bed and keeping your voice to a reasonable level, the nurse should be able to offer as much privacy as required. After introducing yourself to the individual, the nurse should then ensure that the individual provides consent to talk to him or her.

The assessment usually starts with the essential information about the individuals themselves and includes: name, address, date of birth, National Health number, telephone number, next of kin (or who to contact in an emergency) and their contact details, contact details of their general practitioner (GP) and any other health-care professionals involved with the individual, e.g. district nurses, health visitors and physiotherapists.

The form will also require nurses to record information about the individual's occupation, ethnic background, language, religious beliefs and any specific cultural/ethnic requirements.

The next part of the assessment looks at the clinical aspects of the individual – providing a background to the health history to date. The type of information required usually covers the following.

Past medical history (PMH)

- Chronological list of major illnesses, injuries and operations
- Any current diagnosed health problems, e.g. diabetes, asthma or heart disease
- Reason for admission (or referral) – it is important to establish that the individual is aware of the rationale for his or her admission
- Any other health issues.

Medications/drug history

- Prescribed and over the counter (including contraception)
- Any illegal/non-prescribed drugs
- Alternative and complementary therapies
- Known allergies – type of reaction, action taken and outcome.

General

- Alcohol and tobacco consumption
- Dietary preferences

- Food allergies
- Bowel habits
- Mobility – any aids used, e.g. walking stick.

Specific

- Sight: do they wear spectacles or contact lenses?
- Hearing: any aids used?
- Taste: any dentures or bridges?
- Skin: any problems with skin integrity or skin problems?
- Sensory: any deficits in the touch sensation?

Gender related

- Males: any prostate or testicular problems?
- Women: date of last period. Any concerns about menstruation or breast lumps/discharge?

The next section of the assessment requires some observations to be recorded – often referred to as baseline observations. These are essential to provide all health-care professionals with a starting point for the individual's basic biophysical measurements, which provide useful comparisons for future measurements. These measurements are recorded in the care plan or notes and on the relevant observation charts and will always include:

- blood pressure (BP)
- pulse
- respiration
- temperature
- weight
- height
- urinalysis
- other specific observations, e.g. blood sugar and peak flow measurements for individuals with specific known health problems.

This information is comprehensive and initially when nurses start doing an assessment such as the above, it can seem to take forever! However, this is a very useful teaching tool and, with practice, nurses become much more accomplished and efficient at documenting information (Benner 1984). During assessment, the information may come from the individual him- or herself and/or a carer or family member. Information may also be available in the form of patient-held records – such as individuals with specific health problems, e.g. diabetes mellitus, asthma, epilepsy and those taking certain medications. There may also be a referral letter from a doctor or other health-care professional outlining the individual's medical history. The individual may already have a set of medical and/or nursing notes available, but it is always worth checking the details to ensure that the information is factual and accurate.

During the assessment, the nurse has an excellent opportunity to observe the individual both verbally and non-verbally. Obviously a lot of information can be obtained from the verbal responses. However, if the individual continually asks you to repeat the questions, you may conclude he or she has a hearing problem or, if speech is slurred, it might suggest that he or she has had a stroke or some other neurological event.

Just as the verbal responses provide essential information, so the non-verbal (often referred to as 'body language') observations can also be very useful. Observing how an individual responds to questions, whether they appear relaxed, anxious or nervous, can add valuable data to the assessment process.

Other cues may be more subtle – you might note that the skin and lips appear dry, suggesting dehydration. More stoical individuals may not like to admit that they have pain – but appear pale or in obvious discomfort, perhaps holding or rubbing the affected area. In some senses the nurse becomes a detective – searching for clues and looking for evidence to solve what may be a mystery as to the individual's health problem.

There are some special circumstances that nurses encounter during assessment and it is outside the remit of this particular chapter to go through them in detail, but they include:

- individuals who are unconscious
- individuals who do not speak English
- individuals with mental health problems
- individuals with a learning disability/special needs
- babies and children
- aggressive individuals.

In addition to documenting this information in the relevant care plan, any unusual or untoward findings should be reported promptly to the nurse in charge and/or medical team. Once all this information has been recorded, the next stage is planning the care to be delivered.

Planning: how may these needs be met?

During this stage, it is important to establish how the needs or goals of the individual may be met, that these goals are set in order of priority, that the best way of achieving the goals is established and what the alternatives might be.

The care plan allows for individualization at this point, because, although there may be common needs to be met, individuals do respond differently to both disease processes and nursing interventions.

The nurse needs to determine what nursing care will be undertaken to prevent or manage problems. This includes:

- preventing identified potential problems from becoming actual problems
- solving actual problems

- alleviating those problems that cannot be solved and assisting the individual to cope positively with these problems
- preventing recurrence of a treated problem
- helping a person to be as pain-free and comfortable as possible when death is inevitable.

To demonstrate this more clearly, a practical example demonstrates the nursing process and subsequent care plan.

Practical example

Mr Smith is a 76-year-old widower who has been admitted to the ward with a sudden onset of shortness of breath. He had a heart attack 2 years ago and has been taking medication for heart failure for the last 3 months.

Once he is in bed, he has obvious trouble breathing and cannot complete a sentence without gasping for breath. As the nurse admitting Mr Smith, you notice that his ankles are very swollen and his breathing sounds 'bubbly'.

Mr Smith also suffers from diabetes and has not been taking his prescribed tablets in the last 2 days, because of feeling unwell.

The referral letter from his GP, who requested that Mr Smith be admitted to hospital, expressed concern that his house was untidy with little food available.

Immediate problems need to be identified and dealt with urgently, e.g. Mr Smith will need to have his breathing problem dealt with immediately. His symptoms (breathlessness, swollen ankles and bubbly breathing) suggest that he is suffering from heart failure and will need oxygen therapy and medication to help him excrete the excess fluid from his circulatory system, thereby relieving his symptoms.

Less urgent problems can wait – in this example Mr Smith's diabetes may become a cause for concern because he has not been taking the medication regulating his blood sugar. This needs to be dealt with in the next hour or two, but only once his acute breathing problem has been managed effectively.

Other problems – in this case, Mr Smith's potential social problem related to his housing – will require referral to other health-care professionals. Social Services or the intermediate care team should be made aware of Mr Smith's problems so that a better home environment can be established before his discharge from hospital.

At this stage the expected outcomes or results need to be established. Some thought needs to be given to how the individual will benefit from the nursing care. What will the individual be able to achieve and in what time frame?

Mr Smith has initially three identified problems:

1. inability to breathe as a result of heart failure
2. potentially uncontrolled diabetes
3. poor and inadequate housing.

Problem 1 must be dealt with immediately and the administration of prescribed oxygen and a diuretic medication (which speeds up fluid elimination from the body) will rapidly improve his condition.

Problem 2 needs to be addressed within the next hour or two and will involve some initial measurement and observation of his blood sugar levels, with some further health promotion and education on how to manage his diabetes (Katz and Peberdy 1997).

Problem 3 is a long-term problem that will require the input of other health-care professionals. Although this problem is not immediate, it will potentially have an impact on his long-term health, e.g. Mr Smith may find climbing the stairs in his house increasingly difficult if he is out of breath. His shortness of breath may also account for why the house was untidy and little food was evident. He would find it very difficult to walk around his house or go shopping with such shortness of breath.

So each problem here is important and has an effect on his health – but there is clearly a priority or order with which they need to be dealt.

Implementation: what care is actually delivered?

The care plan drawn up now needs to be implemented – there is no point in writing a beautiful care plan if no one actually does anything with it! Nurses also need to keep in mind what they are doing and *why* they are doing it. It is very easy to get carried away with writing and thinking about individuals' problems without relating them back to what is achievable in a given timeframe. Implementation therefore focuses on the actual steps taken to deliver care.

During this stage, nurses should continuously assess the individual's current health status before acting – because some problems do resolve without any intervention or may change dramatically and quickly. Nurses then undertake the care or intervention – perhaps applying a dressing to a wound – and then assess the response. All interventions should be accurately recorded and documented, with any adverse or unexpected outcomes reported immediately. Nurses need to decide what is going to be documented and where. The care plan allows for some free-text writing, so that any additional notes can be added as necessary.

Crucial to this stage (and indeed every stage of the nursing process) are some key assessment skills for considering how the individual is responding to treatment:

- observing
- measuring
- listening
- talking.

Evaluation: have the goals been met?

It may sound obvious, but simply observing the patient can provide you with the answer you need. If we use our example of Mr Smith, the nurse would be *observing* and *measuring* that his breathing or respiratory rate has reduced from 50 breaths/minute to 25 breaths/minute and *listening* to hear that he is able to complete a sentence without getting breathless. These are two simple observations that allow nurses to assess his first problem and determine whether the treatment has been successful. The nurse would also be *talking* to Mr Smith to ask how he is feeling generally.

Nurses should always evaluate their interventions or actions. Evaluation is the part of the cycle when the nurse judges the effectiveness or otherwise of a nursing intervention in terms of the expected outcome (Kemp and Richardson 1994). How does the individual's health and ability compare with the expected outcome? If he or she achieved the stated outcomes, is the person now ready to manage on his or her own and become independent? One of the key features of the nursing process is to encourage individuals to move from total dependence towards total independence. This is not always achievable with every individual, but, on the scale between these two points, the nursing process can assist the individual to achieve a degree of independence, no matter how small that may be.

$$\longleftarrow \text{\rule{6cm}{0.4pt}} \longrightarrow$$

Total dependence   Total independence

Essential in evaluating our interventions is reviewing whether the goals have been achieved and deciding on alternative action if required. This may mean revisiting the beginning of the nursing process, starting with assessment, and beginning again. Nurses need to observe, question, test and measure the activities undertaken so far. These activities are essential to allow the nurse to reflect on the care given and to ask some questions:

* Have the goals been met?
* Was the action appropriate?
* Are new goals required?

As individuals respond differently to illnesses, disease processes and their treatment, it is not always possible to predict that everyone will have similar outcomes, e.g. Mr Smith may not have responded well to the diuretic medication and may have required a further dose before his respiratory rate was reduced. Some diuretic medications have side effects and other drugs have to be given to counteract these effects. Therefore the nurse's assessment of his treatment is vital in providing the doctor with the relevant information to treat his heart failure.

Similarly, for Mr Smith's second problem of potentially uncontrolled diabetes, the plan may have been to provide Mr Smith with more information about his diabetes. In this way we would be encouraging him to develop greater independence in self-managing his diabetes. But we may discover that Mr Smith has a good understanding of his diabetes, but had simply forgotten to take his tablets. This information is therefore a useful base on which to evaluate his care and plan for a different goal.

It is essential that the information about the individual's needs is factual, relevant and comprehensive. Documentation of nursing care is very important and the next section addresses some of the important issues related to documentation and record keeping in general.

Documentation

Documentation of what care has taken place is essential for a number of reasons:

- Communication with others of what has been observed or done
- Identification of roles of individual health-care professionals
- Provision of a record of clinical actions taken
- Organization and dissemination (or sharing) of information with other health-care professionals
- Demonstration of the order of events relating to individual care.

The Nursing and Midwifery Council (NMC) has published a document called *Guidelines for Records and Records Keeping* (2002), which is relevant to all nurses, including students (see website details, page 36). It provides clear guidance on how clinical records, such as care plans, are documented. The key factors that contribute to effective record keeping are:

- Be factual, consistent and accurate
- Write information as soon as possible after an event has occurred, providing current information on the care and condition of the patient/client
- Write clearly and in such a manner that the text cannot be erased
- Write in such a manner that any alterations or additions are dated, timed and signed so that the original entry can still be read clearly
- Records should be accurately dated, timed and signed, with the signature printed alongside the first entry
- Do not include abbreviations, jargon, meaningless phrases, irrelevant speculation and offensive subjective statements
- Records should be readable as photocopies (in black ink, usually)
- Write, wherever possible, with the involvement of the patient/client or carer
- Write in terms that the patient/client can understand
- Write information consecutively
- Identify problems that have arisen and the action taken to rectify them
- Provide clear evidence of the care planned, the decisions made, the care delivered and the information shared.

Individuals now not only have a legal right to see their records, but also increasingly participate in writing them. With regard to documentation, there are legal frameworks that apply to all health-care professionals, including nurses. The Data Protection Act 1984 gives patients/clients access to their computer-held records and provides eight data protection principles. Data should be:

1. Fairly and lawfully processed
2. Processed for limited purposes
3. Adequate, relevant and not excessive
4. Accurate
5. Kept no longer than necessary
6. Processed in accordance with data subject's rights
7. Secure
8. Not transferred to other countries without adequate protection.

In addition, the Access to Health Records Act 1990 gives patients and clients the right of access to manual (paper) records about themselves that were made after 1 November 1991. There are both legal and professional issues to be aware of when compiling care plans.

Nursing care plans

These documents should represent all the nursing activity carried out for individuals wherever they are being nursed. In some clinical areas these may be referred to as Kardexes, patient assessment forms, patient profiles, or nursing notes or history. Whatever the name or format given, what is essential is that the documentation adheres to the NMC guidelines (as outlined above) and as per trust policy, and provide a comprehensive, accurate and holistic overview of the individual in question.

Some areas will have paper records, some will have electronic and some will have a combination of both. Whatever the format, the records should be stored safely and securely. At all times the nurse should ensure that confidential clinical information remains just that – confidential. It should not be shared with any other patients/clients or member of the individual's family unless specifically requested. It should, as far as possible, be written with the individual.

To demonstrate a care plan, we refer back to Mr Smith and document his care in the sample care plan in Table 2.2. In this instance, Roper et al.'s (1993) ALs have been adopted, but any of the conceptual models will have a similar format.

Conclusion

This chapter has focused on the broader perspective of the nursing process and looked at the four key stages of assessment, planning, implementation and evaluation of care with reference to measurement, observation and communications that are essential for the nursing process to work effectively.

Table 2.2 Sample care plan for Mr Smith

| Date: 2 April 2004 | | Nurse: Suzy Smith | |
| Time: 2.40pm | | Ward: 7B Medical Admissions Unit | |

Assess	Plan	Implement	Evaluate
Mr Smith's initial three main problems[a]	**Goals**	**Nursing interventions**	**Outcomes**
Problem 1: breathing – shortness of breath due to probable heart failure	*Problem 1:* • Mr Smith's respiratory rate to decrease from 50 to 25 breaths/min within 2 hours • Mr Smith to be able to complete sentences without getting out of breath within 2 hours	*Problem 1:* • Administer prescribed oxygen and diuretic therapy[b] • Sit Mr Smith upright • Monitor fluid balance • Observe cannula • Document basic observations every 30 min for 4 hours	*Problem 1:* • Respiratory rate now 25 • Continue to monitor basic observations • Ensure Mr Smith has received prescribed ACE inhibitors • Perform ECG
Problem 2: eating and drinking – potential uncontrolled diabetes mellitus	*Problem 2:* • Mr Smith's blood sugar to be maintained within recommended guidelines[c]	*Problem 2:* • Measure and document Mr Smith's blood sugar hourly and urinalysis twice daily	*Problem 2:* • Blood sugar remains elevated • Commence new insulin regimen • Ensure low sugar diet adhered to • Check Mr Smith can monitor his own blood sugar
Problem 3: maintaining a safe environment – poor home environment and potential social issues related to Mr Smith's coping mechanisms at home	*Problem 3:* • Ensure safe home environment on discharge	*Problem 3:* • Call GP • Refer to Social Services • Contact district nurse/intermediate care team	*Problem 3:* • Social worker to visit Mr Smith on ward in 3 days • Liaise with hospital social worker and discharge team

[a]Some areas may have a separate sheet for each problem.
[b]Management of chronic heart failure in primary and secondary care (NICE guideline – see Further information).
[c]Clinical guidelines for type 2 diabetes – management of blood glucose (NICE guideline – see Further information).

Issues related to documentation, both professionally and legally, and a sample care plan have, it is hoped, provided the reader with a clear summary of the nursing process.

There are several advantages of the nursing process. First, its focus is not only on medical problems but also on the human response of individuals. Second, each individual will react differently to medical problems – some will be stoical and others will adopt a 'sick role', taking to their bed at the first hint of a cold or minor illness such as flu. Third, individuals will also respond differently to interventions and their care plans need to reflect this.

Nurses need to take a holistic approach to care. Holism is a term widely used in health care and it refers to the fact that nurses should treat each individual as a whole – taking into account all the ALs – but should not ignore the component parts that contribute towards the individual, or the impacts that society and the environment have on the individual.

Remember Florence Nightingale and her theory of nursing at the beginning? She theorized that a systematic approach to care, which took into account the basic elements of a clean environment, in terms of air, water, light, cleanliness and sanitation, was essential in achieving health and independence. Now, some 150 years later, we continue to use these basic concepts of assessment, planning, implementation and evaluation of care that she used to nurse the soldiers in her care. A wise woman indeed! On a last note, Florence provided advice for nursing students in 1873 by stating:

> Nursing is most truly said to be a high calling, an honourable calling. But what does the honour lie in? In working hard during your training to learn and to do all things perfectly. The honour does not lie in putting on Nursing like your uniform. Honour lies in loving perfection, consistency, and in working hard for it: in being ready to work individually: ready to say not 'How clever I am!' but 'I am not yet worthy; and I will live to deserve to be called a Trained Nurse.
>
> Nightingale (1969)

References

Benner, P. (1984) From Novice to Expert. Excellence and power in clinical nursing practice. Menlo Park, CA: Addison-Wesley.

Chinn, P.L. and Kramer, M.K. (1995) Theory and Nursing: A systematic approach, 4th edn. St Louis, MI: Mosby.

Katz, J. and Peberdy, A. (1997) Promoting Health. Knowledge and practice. Basingstoke: Macmillan Press.

Kemp, N. and Richardson, E. (1994) The Nursing Process and Quality Care. London: Edward Arnold.

McDonald, L. (ed.) (2002) The Collected Works of Florence: An introduction to her life and family. Waterloo, Ontario: Wilfrid Laurier University Press

Neuman, B. (1982) The Neuman Systems Model. Norwalk, CT: Appleton–Century–Crofts.

Nightingale, F. (1969) Notes on Nursing: What it is and what it is not. New York: Dover. (Replication of unabridged 1860 edition.)

Orem, D. (1980) Nursing: Concepts of practice, 2nd edn. New York: McGraw-Hill.

Peplau, H. (1988) Interpersonal Relations in Nursing: A conceptual framework of reference for psychodynamic nursing. Basingstoke: Macmillan Education.

Roper, N., Logan, W. and Tierney, A.J. (1993) The Elements of Nursing: A model for nursing based on a model of living. Edinburgh: Churchill Livingstone.

Roy, C. (1984) Introduction to Nursing: An adaptation model. Englewood Cliffs, NJ: Prentice Hall.

Wilkinson, J. (1996) Nursing Process: A critical thinking approach. Menlo Park, CA: Addison-Wesley.

Further information

Further information on Florence Nightingale can be found at:
www.florence-nightingale.co.uk
www.florence-nightingale-foundation.org.uk
www.spartacus.schoolnet.co.uk/ REnightingale.htm
www.qmuc.ac.uk/hn/history/

Other organizations

Royal College of Nursing (RCN): www.rcn.org.uk
Nursing and Midwifery Council (NMC): www.nmc-org.uk

Nursing and Midwifery Council

An NMC guide for students of nursing and midwifery:
www.nmc-uk.org/nmc/main/publications/2530GuideForStudents.pdf
Code of Professional Conduct
www.nmc-uk.org/nmc/main/publications/codeOfProfessionalConduct.pdf
Guidelines for Records and Records Keeping
www.nmc-uk.org/nmc/main/publications/guidelinesForRecordskeep.pdf

Department of Health

A First Class Service (1998) www.open.gov.uk/doh/newnhs/quality.htm
The NHS Plan (2000) www.doh.gov/nhsplan/default.htm
National Service Frameworks: www.doh.gov.uk/nsf

Careers in nursing

www.learnaboutnursing.org
www.nhscareers.nhs.uk/

National Institute for Clinical Excellence (NICE)

Clinical guidelines for type 2 diabetes – management of blood glucose: www.nice.org.uk/pdf/NICE_full_blood_glucose.pdf
Management of chronic heart failure in primary and secondary care: www.nice.org.uk/pdf/Full_HF_Guideline.pdf

CHAPTER 3

Minimizing health-care-associated risk

JANET G. MIGLIOZZI

'The hospital should do the sick no harm' (Nightingale 1859) and yet patients are harmed when in hospital with 850 000 'adverse events' happening each year – this equates to one in ten patients who are admitted to hospital. Furthermore, adverse events cost the NHS around £3 billion a year in additional hospital stays, health-care-acquired infections and the settlement of negligence claims (Parish 2003).

Maintaining a safe environment in hospitals depends not only on the infrastructure, but also on the equipment and materials used on the premises, and all health-care personnel, irrespective of the setting, are responsible for maintaining a safe environment.

Breaches in safety are often caused by human conduct and can be prevented (Kozier et al. 2000). Consequently, health professionals need to be aware of factors that affect the safety of patients and staff, what constitutes a safe environment for a particular person or a group of people in a health-care setting, and act to minimize risk appropriately.

This chapter considers the minimization of risk to both patients and staff in the health-care setting. The importance of risk assessment and risk minimization is discussed in order to promote safe and effective care. Common risks to health-care staff and patients are then outlined. The second part of the chapter focuses on three areas of practice: drug administration, prevention of falls, and infection prevention and control; it explores methods to minimize risk relating to these themes in the health-care setting.

Risk assessment

As all health care involves risk, and although risk cannot be totally eradicated, health professionals have a duty to ensure that the necessary action is taken to reduce the risk to patients and much can be done to ensure that it is kept to a minimum (Curran 2001). The Health and Safety Executive (HSE 1998) defines a hazard as 'anything that can cause harm' where harm includes injury, ill-health, damage to plant, equipment, property and the environment, and interruption to service delivery (HSE 1997). A risk is the probability that harm will arise, i.e. 'the chance, high or low, that someone will be harmed by the hazard' (HSE 1998) and is therefore, as argued by Mayatt (2002), 'something that can be changed'.

Risk assessment helps to identify and manage workplace hazards that may pose a threat to the health, safety and welfare of people, or to the delivery of care (McCulloch 1999). The HSE (1997) describes risk assessment as a structured process involving five steps:

1. Hazard identification
2. Identification of who might be harmed and how
3. Risk evaluation
4. Documentation of risk assessment
5. Risk assessment review and revision.

Hazard identification

Hazards could result in significant harm under the conditions of the workplace and these would include:

- Slipping/tripping hazards from poorly maintained floors or stairs
- Fire from flammable materials
- Chemicals that are harmful to health, e.g. disinfectants and laboratory solutions
- Electricity, e.g. poor wiring
- Dust
- Fumes
- Manual handling
- Noise
- Poor lighting
- Low or high temperature
- Machinery and equipment used in day-to-day practices.

Identification of who might be harmed and how

- People sharing the workplace
- Operators
- Cleaners
- Office staff
- Members of the public, e.g. visitors
- Staff and patients with disabilities
- Inexperienced staff
- Lone workers.

Risk evaluation

This step includes a consideration of how likely it is that each hazard could cause harm and deciding for each significant hazard whether the risk is high, medium or low, and whether or not the risk has been reduced as far as is reasonably practicable.

Documentation of risk assessment

Written documentation of the precautions to be taken, e.g. guidelines and procedures, should be made. If the risk is not adequately controlled, then an indication of what needs to be done, e.g. an 'action list', should be documented.

Risk assessment review and revision

On review this involves checking that each hazard is still adequately controlled. If not, an indication of the action to be taken must be made.

Key legislation for managing a safe environment is the Health and Safety at Work Act (Department of Health or DoH 1974) which specifies the general duties of employers towards employees and others, including members of the public and patients in health care, and also the duties of employees to themselves and each other.

However, as argued by Mayatt (2002), the Health and Safety at Work Act (DoH 1974) also forms the basis for all other occupational health and safety legislation:

- Health and Safety at Work Act 1974
- Management of Health and Safety at Work Regulations 1999
- Control of Substances Hazardous to Health Regulations (COSHH) 1999
- Manual Handling Operations Regulations 1992
- Display Screen Equipment Regulations 1992
- Personal Protective Equipment Regulations 1992
- Ionising Radiation Regulations 1999
- Electricity at Work Regulations 1989
- Noise at Work Regulations 1989
- Genetically Modified Organisms (Contained Use) Regulations 1992 and 1996 Amendment
- First Aid at Work Regulations 1981
- Consultation with Employees Regulations 1996
- Safety Representative Regulations 1977
- Reporting of Injuries, Diseases and Dangerous Occurrences Regulations (RIDDOR) 1995
- Working Time Regulations 1998
- Provision and Use of Work Equipment Regulations 1998
- Lifting Operations and Lifting Equipment Regulations 1998
- Workplace (Health, Safety and Welfare) Regulations 1992
- Construction (Design and Management) Regulations 1994
- Construction (Health, Safety and Welfare) Regulations 1996
- Control of Asbestos at Work Regulations 1987
- Control of Lead at Work Regulations 1998
- Environmental Protection Act 1990.

Common risks in health care

Individuals employed in health-care settings can be exposed to a broad range of risk that may result in harm. Commonly encountered risks include (Mayatt 2002):

- manual handling
- hazardous chemicals and biological agents
- aggression and violence
- stress
- ionizing and non-ionizing radiation.

Patients in health-care settings are at risk of:

- pressure ulcers
- infection
- falling
- malnutrition
- constipation.

Common factors affecting patient safety

As a result of illness or disability, certain groups of patients are unable to protect themselves and are inherently more at risk of injury (Table 3.1).

Table 3.1 Factors affecting patient safety

Age and development	The risk of injury will vary with age and level of development, e.g. young and elderly people are particularly vulnerable
Sensory perception	Individuals with impaired hearing, sight, touch, smell and touch perception are highly susceptible to injury, particularly in a strange environment
Cognitive awareness	Impaired/altered awareness caused by confusion, disease, medication or impaired level of consciousness increase the risk of injury
Ability to communicate	A diminished ability to receive and convey information is a risk for injury as the individual is unable to interpret or read information
Mobility and health status	Individuals with poor mobility or impaired coordination are more at risk of injury
Safety awareness	Information is crucial to safety, particularly for an individual in an unfamiliar environment
Emotional state	Stress can alter an individual's ability to concentrate and decrease awareness of environmental hazards

Adapted from Kozier et al. (2000).

Minimizing the risk of medication error

'The administration of medicines is an important aspect of the professional practice of persons whose names are on the Council's register' (NMC, 2002b). Medication errors are consistently reported to account for between 10 and 20% of all adverse events (DoH 2001a) with 10 000 serious adverse drug reactions reported each year in the UK (DoH 2000a). Furthermore, 4–10% of prescriptions are illegible or ambiguous (DoH 2000a). Illegible prescriptions are also a major cause of medication error as the reader is forced to make his or her own interpretation of the prescription and this places the patient at risk. The prescription should always be clear, unambiguous and leave no doubt as to the prescriber's intentions (DoH 2001a).

Errors can arise in drug selection, prescribing, dispensing, administration and therapeutic monitoring (Fijin 2002). The most common types of errors are giving the wrong drug or wrong dose, using the wrong route and failing to check the patient's identity (O'Shea 1999).

In 2001, the Department of Health set out specific action to be taken in relation to medication error with the aim being to reduce serious errors in the use of prescribed drugs by 40%.

In seeking to minimize the risk of medication error and ensure patients' safety the following steps should be adhered to (adapted from Hogston and Simpson 2002).

The right medication

The label of the container should be checked against the prescription chart to ensure that it is the correct prescribed medication and medication should be dispensed only from the original container. Any instructions pertaining to the medication and the expiry date should also be noted. The person dispensing the drug should be familiar with basic information about the drug, its action, any contraindications and side effects.

The right patient

Before dispensing the medication, it is important to check that the right patient is receiving it. Checking the patient's identification bracelet and asking him or her to state his or her name are two ways of doing this.

The right time

To maintain a constant blood plasma level of the drug at an effective range, it is important to give the drug as close to the prescribed time as possible. Similarly, certain drugs need to be given before, with or after a meal in order to maximize the drug's effect, so it is important that this is adhered to and that an explanation is given to the patient to ensure compliance with the drug regimen.

The right dose

When drugs are prescribed at different strengths to that required, it is important that the right amount of drug is calculated and this will require a basic knowledge of arithmetic. Similarly, a calibrated medicine pot or syringe may be required for liquid medications/injectable preparations. Where the dose to be given is in doubt or a complicated calculation is required, this should be double-checked with another health professional.

The right route

Drugs may be administered in a number of ways including by mouth, rectally, via injection intramuscularly or intravenously, topically or via inhalation, although not all the drugs can be administered by all the possible routes. Indeed, some medications can prove fatal if given via the wrong route. Therefore it is important to check the route before administration.

Minimizing the risk of falls

The National Service Framework (NSF) for Older People identifies fall prevention as a priority, as stated in key standard 6 (DoH 2001b). Death, injury, increased dependency and impaired self-care are possible physical consequences of a fall; the psychological effects can also be profound (Downton 1993). There is an increasing risk of falling with increasing age and falls are the leading cause of death from injury among the over-75 age group (Sowden and Dickson 1996), with over 14 000 deaths each year as a result of an osteoporotic hip fracture (DoH 2001b). Factors contributing to increased risk of falling, as identified in the literature (Galloway 1999), can be divided into two groups: intrinsic, i.e. a particular characteristic of the individual, and extrinsic, i.e. an external characteristic (Table 3.2).

Assessing an individual's risk of falling and implementing an appropriate plan of care to reduce the risk is 'preferable to waiting until they fall to take action' (Galloway 1999). Therefore, an assessment of the risk of falling is an essential part of safe practice. Cannard (1996) developed the Fall Risk Assessment Scale for the Elderly (FRASE) and this provides an easy and quick tool for assessment (Table 3.3) which can then be used in conjunction with the individual patient's care plan.

The following are practical interventions that may reduce the risk of falls for elderly patients in a health-care setting (Galloway 1999):

- An appropriate level of supervision
- A means of calling for assistance, e.g. patient call bell
- Addressing the patient's individual elimination needs and ensuring that a urinal or commode (if needed) is available at the bedside at night
- Adequate lighting
- Appropriate and well-fitting footwear

Table 3.2 Characteristics associated with increased risk of falling

Intrinsic characteristics	
Age	Patients in the over-75 age group are the most at risk of falling
History of previous falls	Patients who have fallen once are more likely to fall again (Rogers 1994)
Gender	Men are more likely to fall; however, women who fall are likely to sustain a more serious injury, e.g. hip fracture (Rawsky 1998)
Cognitive/visual/mobility impairment	Specific physical and psychological issues can make an individual patient more at risk of falls (Morse 1997)
Incontinence/urgency	30–34.5% of elderly patients fall when getting up to use the toilet (Bakarich et al. 1997)
Extrinsic characteristics	
Drugs	Certain groups of prescription drugs have been associated with increased risk of falling, e.g. sedatives, analgesics, laxatives and diuretics, hypnotics, tranquillizers and anti-depressants (Effective Healthcare Bulletin 1996)
Environmental hazards	Between a third and a half of falls among elderly people occur as a result of environmental hazard and include: poor lighting, ill-fitting shoes, poorly maintained flooring, e.g. loose carpets/rugs (Effective Healthcare Bulletin 1996)

- Keeping the patient's essential items (drink, spectacles, tissues) within easy reach
- Keeping the bed height at the lowest level
- Using a chair of an appropriate design and height for the patient.

Minimizing the risk of health-care-acquired infection

In health care there are infection risks for both patients and staff (McCulloch 1999) and, in order to minimize these risks, principles of infection prevention and control must be implemented and adhered to by all concerned. Therefore, in seeking to reduce the risk of health-care-acquired infection, both environmental and clinical factors need to be considered (Figure 3.1).

Environmental factors

The infection hazards associated with the actual environment in which patients are nursed are often overlooked (Parker 1999a); however, the importance of the environment to the well-being of the patient should not be

Table 3.3 Fall Risk Assessment Scale for the Elderly (FRASE) (Cannard 1996)

Risk factor	Score	Action (total score)
Male 1		3–8 = low risk
Female 2		9–12 = medium risk
Age		13+ = high risk
60–70	1	
71–80	2	
81+	1	
Gait		
Steady	0	
Hesitant	1	
Poor transfer	3	
Unsteady	3	
Sensory deficit		
Sight	2	
Hearing	1	If score > 1 for mobility/gait, sensory deficit
Balance	2	or medication, refer to
Falls history		physiotherapy/occupational
None	0	therapy/medical staff as appropriate
At home	2	
In ward	1	
Both	3	
Medication		
Hypnotics	1	
Tranquillizers	1	
Hypotensives	1	
Mobility		
Full	1	
Uses aid	2	
Restricted	3	
Bed bound	1	
Medical history		
Diabetes	1	
Dementia/confusion	1	
Fits	1	

ignored. Furthermore, dirty hospital environments have been implicated in outbreaks of infection (Ayliffe et al. 1990), in particular outbreaks caused by enteric viruses (Green et al. 1998). Since the launch of *The NHS Plan* (DoH 2000b), national investment to improve the cleanliness, tidiness and appearance of hospitals has been implemented. Similarly, national cleaning standards for hospitals have been developed (DoH 2001c).

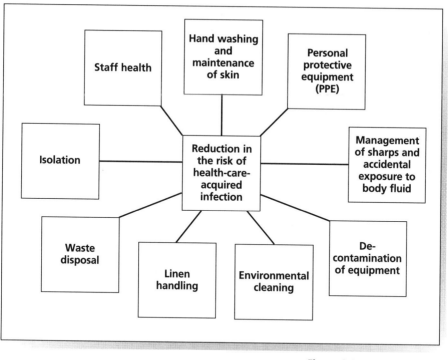

Figure 3.1
Key infection control principles
to reduce the risk of health-
care-acquired infection.

Environmental cleaning

Any health-care environment presents an infection risk to patients and staff because dust, soil and organic matter, which are potentially infectious, quickly accumulate in the environment if it is not properly and regularly cleaned. Cleaning procedures should concentrate on areas with greater environmental risk, such as toilets, patients' beds and lockers and kitchens, and thorough cleaning can prevent the spread of micro-organisms such as methicillin-resistant *Staphylococcus aureus* (MRSA) (DoH 1996).

Therefore, cleaning the health-care environment is a cost-effective way of controlling infection (Chadwick and Oppenheim 1996). Cleaning the environment has two purposes (Parker 1999a):

1. To improve/restore the appearance, maintain function and prevent deterioration
2. To reduce the number of microbes present and remove substances that will support their growth or interfere with subsequent disinfection or sterilization processes.

Cleaning involves the use of detergent and water to remove organic material and micro-organisms, and approximately 80% of micro-organisms are removed during the cleaning process (Gaze 1990). It is not necessary to use disinfectants for general cleaning because their effect is short-lived (Gaze 1990); nevertheless, disinfectant granules should be used to remove spills of body fluids because they will destroy the micro-organisms present and thus reduce the risk of infection to the person clearing up the spillage (UK Health Departments 1998). However, disinfectant granules should not be used on urine spills, because an irritant chlorine vapour may be released (DoH 1990). The use of a disinfectant after cleaning is recommended where there is a high level of environmental contamination, e.g. during an outbreak of infection (Noble et al. 1998), although care should be taken with its use near fabrics or carpet as disinfectant granules will damage these materials (Wilson 2001). Equipment used for cleaning, e.g. mops and buckets, should be decontaminated and stored dry to prevent multiplication of micro-organisms.

Decontamination of equipment

Confusion often surrounds the decontamination of equipment used in health care and the decision to clean, disinfect or sterilize depends on the risk of the equipment transmitting infection or acting as a source of infection (Wilson 2001). Decontamination is a general term meaning the process of removing microbial material and an outline of the aims of the different levels of decontamination is given in Table 3.4. Risk assessment can be used to select the appropriate method of decontamination and Table 3.5 provides an indication of the level of decontamination required depending on the risk of the item used.

Table 3.4 Aims of different levels of decontamination (Ayliffe et al. 1992)

Method	Aim
Sterilization	Removes or destroys all micro-organisms including spores
Disinfection	Reduces the number of micro-organisms to a level at which they are not harmful; spores are not usually destroyed
Cleaning	Physical removal of contamination and many micro-organisms

Waste disposal

The NHS has a legal responsibility for the safe disposal of hazardous waste that is regulated by the Environmental Protection Act 1990 and the Environmental Protection Regulations 1991. As hospital waste can harbour micro-organisms and is therefore potentially harmful to staff, patients, the public and the environment (Wilson 2001), in order to minimize risk it is important that all waste is properly segregated according to type (Table 3.6) and discarded in the appropriate colour-coded bag to ensure the correct method of disposal (Table 3.7).

Table 3.5 Categories of risk and level of decontamination required (Ayliffe et al. 1992)

Category	Indication	Examples	Decontamination process	Methods
High risk	Items that penetrate the skin or mucous membranes, or enter sterile body areas	Surgical instruments, needles	Sterilization	Autoclave or sterile single-use disposable
Medium risk	Items that have contact with mucous membranes or are contaminated by microbes that are easily transmitted	Endoscopes, bedpans, vaginal specula	Disinfection or sterilization	Chemically disinfect Pasteurize Autoclave
Low risk	Items used on intact skin	Mattresses, washbowls, floors	Cleaning	Wash with detergent and hot water and dry

Table 3.6 Classification of waste

Domestic waste	Clinical waste	Sharps waste	Waste for autoclaving	Non-infectious human waste
Household waste, e.g. paper, flowers, food	Material contaminated with blood or body fluid, human or animal tissue	Needles, syringes, broken glass and other contaminated sharp items	Pathology specimens	Sanitary towels, incontinence pads

Table 3.7 Colour coding for the disposal of health-care waste (Health Services Advisory Committee 1999)

Type of waste	Colour of bag/container	Method of disposal
Domestic	Black bag	Landfill
Clinical	Yellow bag	Incineration
Sharps	Yellow sharps containers	Incineration
Pathology	Blue or transparent with blue inscription	Autoclave and then landfill
Non-infectious human	Yellow, black stripes	Landfill

Linen handling

Used linen is a potential infection risk, especially if it is contaminated with body fluids or has been used in the care of a patient with an infectious disease. Linen used by the health service must be washed at the highest possible temperature and dried quickly to ensure that micro-organisms are destroyed (McCulloch 1999). Guidelines for the management of used or infected linen (NHS Executive 1995) state that laundries that process hospital linen must comply with Department of Health guidance on disinfection, staff protection and effluent control in order to minimize the risks of personal contamination when handling used linen. Consequently, laundering at a ward level is not advised because most health-care settings are not able to comply with Department of Health guidance as there is no safe means of monitoring control measures.

In minimizing risk from used linen, guidelines for the safe handling of linen include the following (adapted from Barrie 1994):

- Wear a plastic apron for bed making.
- When handling contaminated linen, gloves and plastic apron should be worn and hands washed after contact.
- Linen that is contaminated with body fluid should be placed, first, into a dissolvable liner, secured tightly and then placed into an appropriate linen bag.
- Linen should be bagged at the bedside.
- Use the national colour coding system (Table 3.8).
- Securely fasten the linen bag when full.

Table 3.8 outlines the national colour coding system for the segregation of used linen into linen skips/containers.

Table 3.8 National colour coding system for hospital linen

Category	Bag colour	Description
Used	White linen or plastic	Used, soiled and foul linen
Infected	Water-soluble bag with red outer linen or plastic bag	Linen used by patients who have an infectious disease
Heat labile	White with an orange stripe	Fabrics that are likely to be damaged by a hot wash

Management of sharps and accidental exposure to body fluid

'Sharps' include needles, scalpels, broken glass or other items that may cause a laceration or puncture and may be contaminated with body fluid. Sharp instruments frequently cause injury to health-care workers (Wilson 2001) and the main hazards of a sharps injury are hepatitis B, hepatitis C and HIV. There were 1550 reports of blood-borne virus exposure in health-care workers between July 1997 and June 2002 (Royal College of Nursing 2004). Accidental exposure to body fluids can occur by:

- percutaneous injury, e.g. needlestick injury
- exposure of broken skin
- exposure of mucous membranes.

The reporting of injuries and dangerous diseases regulations (RIDDOR) impose a duty of care on the employer to report certain types of incident to the Health and Safety Executive (HSE 1995) and this includes sharps injuries and accidental exposure to blood-borne viruses.

However, the risk of a sharps injury can be minimized by adhering to safe practice when using or disposing of sharps and complying with COSHH regulations:

- Wear appropriate personal protective equipment
- Assemble devices with care
- Do not re-sheathe needles unless unavoidable, in which case a commercial re-sheathing device should be used
- Do not carry used sharps by hand or pass to another person
- Do not disassemble sharp before disposal – discard as one unit
- Discard used sharp in a sharps box that complies with UN3291 and BS7320 standards
- Take sharps box to the point of use to enable immediate disposal
- Ensure sharps boxes are available at all locations where sharps are used
- Sharps boxes should be placed on a level surface or wall mounted below shoulder height
- Close the sharps box aperture between use
- Never overfill sharps boxes – adhere to the 'fill to' line
- Lock sharps box when full
- Do not place sharps boxes into clinical waste bags

Figure 3.2 shows the steps that the nurse should take following accidental exposure to body fluids.

Personal protective equipment

The correct use of personal protective equipment (PPE) is an essential component of safe practice and the minimization of hazard exposure. Within the context of infection control PPE includes:

- disposable gloves
- disposable aprons

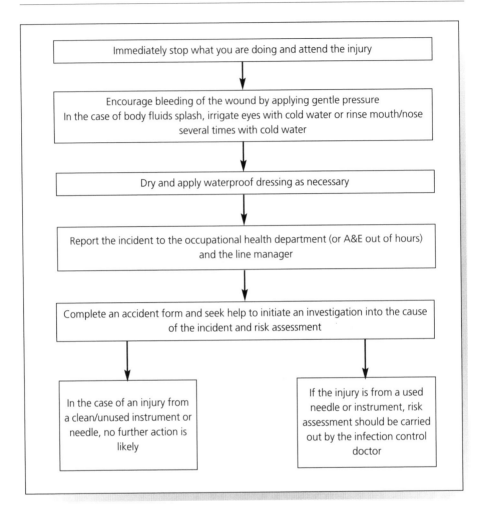

Figure 3.2
Actions to take following accidental
exposure to body fluid. (Adapted
from Royal College of Nursing 2004.)

- eye protection
- mouth protection
- food protection
- fluid-repellent gowns.

The type of protective clothing chosen for use should be based on a risk assessment of the possible risk of contamination, rather than the infection encountered. Similarly, the principle of routine infection control (or universal) precautions requires that staff take precautions to protect themselves from contact with any potentially infectious substances encountered during the course of their work and there must be a readily available supply of the types of protective clothing that are likely to be required (McCulloch 1999).

Routine infection control (universal) precautions (Wilson 2001)

Hand washing

- Before and after contact with patients
- After gloves are removed
- After contact with body fluids

Maintain skin integrity

- Cover cuts with waterproof dressing
- Dry skin properly and use handcream

Protective clothing

- Use to protect against direct contact with body fluid
- Assess risk of procedure and select appropriate protection

Sharps safety

- Use equipment with safety devices
- Use safe handling and disposal procedures
- Provide hepatitis B immunization for staff at risk
- Report exposure to blood or body fluid

Safe handling of clinical waste

- Use safe handling and disposal procedure
- Discard excreta directly into drainage system
- Incinerate contaminated disposable material

Decontamination of equipment

- Clean and decontaminate equipment after use
- Disinfect used linen by laundering
- Use protective clothing while handling and cleaning

Decontamination of environment

- Keep environment clean and free from dust
- Disinfect spills of body fluid

Isolation

The aim of isolation is to minimize the risk of micro-organisms from the affected person being transferred to others (known as source isolation – formerly barrier nursing) or to prevent the spread of infection to a patient who has reduced resistance to infection (protective isolation – formerly known as reverse barrier nursing). Isolation procedures are the outcome of a risk assessment, which includes the source of infection, route of transmission (see below) and the susceptibility of others (Parker 1999b); the principle of isolation is to isolate the micro-organism not the patient (Wilson 2001).

Physical segregation from other patients is particularly recommended where an infection is transmitted by airborne particles or respiratory droplets, or there is likely to be gross contamination of the environment, e.g. if a patient has profuse diarrhoea.

Routes for possible transmission of micro-organisms

Contact: the most common route of transmission of infection is via direct (person to person) or indirect (instruments or equipment) contact.

Respiratory: the infection is spread via respiratory secretions generated by coughing and sneezing.

Airborne: micro-organisms are transferred by droplet nuclei (minute particles) or by dust particles. Air currents will carry these particles and disperse them in the environment.

Food or waterborne: some infections can be transmitted via the ingestion of contaminated food or water, resulting in gastrointestinal symptoms.

Vector borne: diseases can be transmitted by vectors such as lice, mosquitoes and ticks.

Staff health

Health-care workers have always been at risk of both acquiring and transmitting infection (May 2000). Access to an occupational health service should be available to all staff working in health care and, to minimize the risk of occupational exposure, guidelines for safe practice include (May 2000):

* covering lesions on hands with waterproof dressings
* appropriate management of skin conditions, e.g. psoriasis, eczema
* immunization, e.g. hepatitis B, rubella
* pre-employment health screening
* reporting of accidents and adverse events
* restriction of non-immune/pregnant staff in certain situations
* counselling and support.

Hand washing

The hands of health-care personnel are the most common vehicle by which micro-organisms are transmitted between patients, and hands are frequently implicated as the route of transmission in outbreaks of infection (Wilson 2001). Hand washing is a simple but effective means of protecting patients from infections (Kerr 1998). Furthermore, as each health-care professional has a duty to promote and safeguard the interests of patients, identify the risks and take the appropriate action to minimize them (NMC 2002a), hand hygiene is paramount.

In most care settings, hand washing with liquid soap and water is adequate. However, when caring for patients in isolation or if a greater level of skin decontamination is required, e.g. before undertaking surgery/sterile procedures, then one of the following antiseptic aqueous solutions should be used (adapted from Parker 1999c).

Chlorhexidine gluconate

A broad-spectrum antiseptic that has a residual effect on the skin and remains active for several hours, and so is ideal for a surgical scrub.

Iodophors

Iodine is an excellent antiseptic agent; however, it can be irritating to the skin and cause staining. It has a broad spectrum of activity but is slow acting with minimal residual activity.

Alcohols

These are fast acting with rapid reduction of microbial counts and are effective against a broad range of micro-organisms. Alcohols are not good cleaning agents, so visibly soiled hands should be washed with soap and water before using an alcohol hand rub.

Triclosan

This is an effective agent against MRSA, because of its residual activity on the skin.

Alcohol hand rubs and gels

Alcohol is an effective alternative when water or towels are not available and is also useful for rapid hand disinfection (Infection Control Nurses' Association or ICNA 1998) when hands are not visibly soiled.

Hand decontamination technique

Ayliffe et al. (1992) make the point that hand washing that is performed at the right time using a good technique, where all surfaces of the hands are covered, is more important than the agent used or length of time of hand washing, and hands should be washed for 10–15 seconds (Larson 1995). The indications for hand decontamination are:

- before starting work
- before any aseptic or invasive procedure
- after prolonged contact with any patient
- after handling any item that is or may be soiled with body fluid
- before handling food
- as soon as hands become visibly soiled
- after removal of gloves
- before contact with any immunosuppressed patients
- before and after entering or leaving source isolation rooms
- on leaving work.

Drying hands thoroughly is also important because damp hands transfer bacteria more readily than dry ones and can become chapped and sore (Gould 1994). Paper hand towels rather than hot air dryers should be used; however, care must be taken on disposal of these because recontamination of hands can occur if disposal bins do not have foot-operated pedals.

Conclusion

This chapter has explored the importance of risk assessment to the promotion of patient and staff safety, and measures to minimize risk relating to three areas of practice. Maintaining a safe environment will impinge on all aspects of patient care.

The nurse must consider both the safety of the patient and his or her own safety. Minimizing risk should be paramount in all care settings – community and institutional.

Risk assessment can help to identify and prevent risk or harm occurring. The nurse owes a duty of care to the patient and that duty of care will encapsulate safe nursing practice. Each registered nurse must remember that he or she is accountable for his or her actions or omissions.

References

Ayliffe, G.A.J., Collins, B.J. and Taylor L.J. (1990) Hospital Acquired Infection: Principles and practices, 2nd edn. London: Butterworths.

Ayliffe, A.J., Lowbury, E.J.L., Geddes, A.M. and Williams, J.D. (1992) Control of Hospital Infection: A practical handbook, 3rd edn. London: Chapman & Hall Medical.

Bakarich, A., McMillan, V. and Prosser, R. (1997) The effect of nursing intervention on the incidence of older patient falls. Australian Journal of Advanced Nursing 15(1): 26–30.

Barrie, D. (1994) How hospital linen and laundry services are provided. Journal of Hospital Infection 27: 219–235

Cannard, G. (1996) Falling trend. Nursing Times 92(2): 36–37.

Chadwick, C. and Oppenheim, B.A. (1996) Cleaning as a cost-effective method of infection control. The Lancet 347: 1776.

Curran, E. (2001) Reducing the risk of healthcare-acquired infection. Nursing Standard 16(1): 45–52

Department of Health (1974) Health and Safety at Work Act. London: HMSO.

Department of Health (1990) Spills of urine: potential risk of misuse of chlorine-releasing disinfecting agents. Safety Advice Bulletin 59(90): 41.

Department of Health (1996) MRSA: What nursing and residential homes need to know. London: DoH.

Department of Health (2000a) An Organisation with a Memory: Report of an Expert Group on Learning from Adverse Events in the NHS. London: HMSO.

Department of Health (2000b) The NHS Plan. London: HMSO.

Department of Health (2001a) Building a Safer NHS for Patients: Improving medication safety. London: HMSO.

Department of Health (2001b) National Service Framework for Older People. London: HMSO.

Department of Health (2001c) National Cleaning Standards for Hospitals. London: HMSO.

Downton, J.H. (1993) Falls in the Elderly. London: Edward Arnold.

Effective Healthcare Bulletin (1996) Preventing Falls and Subsequent Injury in Older People. Edinburgh: Churchill Livingstone.

Fijin, R. (2002) Hospital prescribing errors: epidemiological assessment of the predictors. British Journal of Clinical Pharmacology 53: 326–332.

Galloway, J. (1999) Risk management of falls for older adults. Nursing and Residential Care 1(1): 20–23.

Gaze, H. (1990) Dirt in hospital: sweeping change? Nursing Times 86(24): 27–28.

Gould, D.J. (1994) Nurses' hand decontamination practice: results of a local study. Journal of Hospital Infection 28: 1530.

Green, J., Wright, P.A. and Gallimore, C.L. (1998) The role of environmental contamination with small round structured viruses in a hospital outbreak investigated by reverse-transcriptase polymerase chain reaction assay. Journal of Hospital Infection 39: 39–45.

Health and Safety Executive (1995) A Guide to the Reporting of Injuries, Diseases and Dangerous Occurrences Regulations. London: HSE.

Health and Safety Executive (1997) Successful Health and Safety Management. London: HSE.

Health and Safety Executive (1998) Five Steps to Risk Assessment. London: HSE.

Health Services Advisory Committee (1999) Safe Disposal of Clinical Waste. Sudbury: HSE Books.

Hogston, R. and Simpson, P.M. (2002) Foundations of Nursing Practice, 2nd edn. Basingstoke: Palgrave Macmillan.

Infection Control Nurses' Association (1998) Guidelines for Hand Hygiene. London: ICNA.

Kerr, J. (1998) Handwashing. Nursing Standard 12(51): 35–39.

Kozier, B., Erb, G., Berman, A.J. and Burke, K. (2000) Fundamentals of Nursing: Concepts, process and practice. Englewood Cliffs, NJ: Prentice Hall Health.

Larson, E. (1995) APIC guidelines for infection control practice. American Journal of Infection Control 23: 251–269.

McCulloch, J. (1999) Risk management in infection control. Nursing Standard 13(34): 44–46.

May, D. (2000) Infection control. Nursing Standard 14(28): 51–57.

Mayatt, V.L. (2002) Managing Risk in Healthcare: Law and practice. London: Butterworths Tolley.

Morse, J. (1997) Preventing Patient Falls. London: Sage.

NHS Executive (1995) Hospital Laundry Arrangements for Used and Infected Linen HSG(95)18. London: HMSO.

Nightingale, F. (1859) Notes on Nursing. Revised, with additions. London: Baillière Tindall.

Noble, M.A., Isaac-Renton, J.L. and Boyce, D.L. (1998) The toilet as a transmission vector of vancomycin-resistant enterococci. Journal of Hospital Infection 40: 237–241.

Nursing and Midwifery Council (2002a) Code of Professional Conduct. London: NMC.

Nursing and Midwifery Council (2002b) Guidelines for the Administration of Medicines. London: NMC.

O'Shea, E. (1999) Factors contributing to medication errors: a literature review. Journal of Clinical Nursing 8: 496–503.

Parish, C. (2003) Make no mistake. Nursing Standard 17(29): 12–13.

Parker, L.J. (1999a) Managing and maintaining a safe environment in the hospital setting. www.internurese.com/cgi-bin/go.pl/library/article.cgi?uid = 6510 (accessed 01/07/04).

Parker, L.J. (1999b) Current recommendations for isolation practices in nursing. British Journal of Nursing 8: 881–887.

Parker, L.J. (1999c) Importance of handwashing in the prevention of cross-infection www.internurse.com/cgi-bin/go.pl/library/article/cgi?uid 6586 (accessed 01/07/04).

Rawsky, E. (1998) Review of the literature on falls among the elderly. Journal of Nursing Scholarship 30(1): 47–52.

Rogers, S. (1994) Reducing falls in a rehabilitation setting: a safer environment through team effort. Rehabilitation Nursing 19: 274–276.

Royal College of Nursing (2004) Working Well Initiative: Good practice in infection control. London: RCN.

Sowden, A. and Dickson, R. (1996) Preventing falls and further injury in older people. Nursing Standard 10(47): 32–33.

UK Health Departments (1998) Guidance for Clinical Health Care Workers: Protection against infection with blood-borne viruses. Recommendations of the Expert Advisory Group on AIDS and the Advisory Group on Hepatitis. London: DoH.

Wilson, J. (2001) Infection Control in Clinical Practice, 2nd edn. London: Baillière Tindall.

CHAPTER 4

Communication and interpersonal skills in nursing

DAVID JOHN BRIGGS

Communication is the process of conveying information between two or more people (Maxim and Bryan 1995). It is impossible to care for someone without exchanging facts or opinions. Whatever path in nursing you may eventually take, you will very quickly have to demonstrate that you can communicate with patients, relatives and other health-care professionals. Communication and interpersonal skills are separate concepts. Individuals cannot communicate without using (good or bad) interpersonal skills. The use of good interpersonal skills is an ability that people, including health-care staff, need to learn. It could be suggested that nurses are experts in communication and interpersonal skills because, without them, it would not be possible to care for people.

For these reasons the chapter starts with the assumption that communication and interpersonal skills are essential for nursing care. The reader is given the opportunity to consider verbal communication skills. In contrast, the next section looks at non-verbal communication, and these two concepts together offer the reader the chance to assimilate some very important aspects of the subject of communication. Interpersonal skills are of a much broader nature than those of communication and a rationale for this assumption is offered. Finally, an insight into a reflection (defined by Boyd and Fales [1983] as the process of internally examining and exploring an issue of concern, triggered by an experience) is offered as a method of learning from situations involving communication and interpersonal skills. The very concepts that are highlighted in the early part of the chapter as important areas for learning are revisited in reflection to ascertain how they may be used in practice. The chapter ends by suggesting that learning in communication and interpersonal skills can be internalized and enhanced through methods of reflection.

Verbal communication

The adjective 'verbal' suggests that communication is linguistic, i.e. spoken, said or unwritten. Effective verbal communication relies on issues such as the tone and the pitch of a person's voice, but equally the use of language will be paramount to attaining an understanding between the giver and the receiver of the message. Expression of speech then becomes important and everyday statements, through slang, sayings, clichés and conventional expressions, form a large part of a speaker's competence (Siditis 2004). Although verbal communication can be effective on its own (e.g. in the use of the telephone), it is important to bear in mind that non-verbal communication reinforces the message given in speech (Ellis 1992). Consequently, in order to be effective, a message presented through just a verbal means of transmission has to be much clearer than one that is sent with the aid of other means of communication.

For speech to enhance this transmission process, the language needs to be clearly recognizable in the basic sounds that the person uses. These sounds are combined to make up words and phrases (phonological grammar). However, the message will have lexical content (what is said) and non-lexical content (how it is said). The lexical part of the message may or may not be clear to the patient and how it is said can enhance the message or reduce its meaning for the recipient. An example of this phenomenon is a patient who asks the student nurse her views on what the food in the hospital is like. In reply the student nurse says 'good' and says it in a cheerful voice. The patient is likely to be reassured that the food will be all right. On the other hand, a student nurse who says 'good' but in a quiet hesitant voice may raise concerns in the patient about the prospect for his or her future nourishment.

Morrison and Burnard (1991) suggest that information can be obtained through the use of a closed question (one that requires a yes or no answer) or one that requires a more open question (one that allows the recipient to offer a full range of replies). The student nurse who works in a primary health-care setting and asks the patient if he or she can return the following morning at 11 o'clock to take the patient's blood pressure is using an example of a closed question. The student nurse could ask the patient how he or she feels about being visited the next morning, and this would allow the patient to offer a range of replies, e.g. the patient may agree to be visited the next day but the time may not be convenient because the gasman is calling. By answering this open-ended question the patient will give the information that he or she believes is important and that he or she would like us to know. However, a closed question can be used very effectively to clarify aspects of an open answer. A yes or no answer can allow the situation to become much clearer, together with meanings that patients attach to events.

Many factors related to the particular situation can also affect how the message is transferred from the receiver to the giver (Porritt 1990). These include the attitudes of both people – the sender and the receiver – and their experiences in coming to the situation, the expectations of both sender and receiver about the other person, and what they thought the outcome of the communication would be. Importantly, both parties may have a hidden agenda within the message. Communication reflects:

- attitudes
- experience
- education and training
- expectations from other people
- hidden agendas
- what a person wants from the outcome of the message.

Health professionals can control the patient encounter partly through the use of language, e.g. the nurse who starts to make arrangements for the next visit is suggesting that she has to leave and the visit is almost at an end. The health professional may set the agenda and lead the conversation by stating the important issues at the start of the interaction; this gives the health professional the ability to hold a level of power over the conversant, once the conversation centres on his or her predetermined topics. There is an element of control in structuring the discussion around areas that the person sees as important. Just as a recipient can be empowered through an open and flexible agenda for discussion, he or she can be disempowered by a hidden agenda and an inflexible form of conversation.

The use of language and conversation may be different according to the gender of the parties involved in the conversation, e.g. research has shown that women perform better than men in tests of remembering what is said (Kimura and Seal 2003). However, it is often assumed that older people cannot remember words or understand phrases so easily. A study by Rodriguez-Aranda (2003) suggests that they cannot coordinate thinking and speech in the way they did when younger. Words chosen carefully by a health professional can enhance the care of a well woman who is attending an antenatal class or the recovery of an elderly patient who is very frail physically.

Non-verbal communication (including listening)

This type of communication involves professionals using their bodies, with the exception of speech, to interact with patients effectively. Non-verbal behaviours include patient-directed eye gaze, head nodding, smiling, forward leaning and touch (Caris-Verhallen et al. 1999). This section considers how non-verbal communication is used as a tool in interactions with patients, how active listening skills can be developed and finally how touch and personality can affect communication with patients.

What does the recipient look at in the non-verbal aspects of the interaction?

Skilled nurses use their body as a tool in their nursing repertoire. Shakespeare (2003) suggests four terms for the way nurses use their bodies: instrumental, corporate, relational and human.

Instrumental

This term suggests that the body movements carried out by the nurse will be much more effective if they are relevant to the instructions that have been given to the patient by the health professional. An example of being instrumental is when a patient is directed to a health visitor's room in a clinic; this is done by pointing to the door in line with her or his instruction.

Corporate

The next is 'corporate' and an example is the effect that wearing a uniform can have on a situation. The uniform may automatically suggest to the patient that the person wearing it has certain skills, which the patient does not have, and as a result he or she may have certain responsibilities to the patient, including a duty of care.

Relational

A further use that the nurse makes of her body is termed 'relational'. The outcomes of care demand that there is a good relationship between the nurse and the patient. Good non-verbal communication, when it is congruent and consistent with what the nurse is saying, can help develop a good rapport between the two people.

Human

The final term, 'human', suggests that humans have the ability to influence the non-verbal use of their bodies, but this may differ as a result of human factors such as gender and being healthy. The use of this influence in an effective manner can enhance the ability to communicate. An example is the use of personal space; some patients may not like people sitting too close to them during a discussion whereas others would prefer the health professional being closer so that they can hear. As Shakespeare (2003) suggests, over a period of time these skills can become automatic, but they can also become taken for granted by the nurse concerned.

The importance of listening

An important area of non-verbal communication that is currently being researched is listening, and Fredrickson (1999) suggests that a nurse uses this key non-verbal skill. Morrison and Burnard (1991) suggest that there are three levels of listening. The first concerns the recipient of the message paying careful attention to the words and phrases that are sent by the person who is delivering them. The second concerns the aspects of the communication such as the accents of the sender of the message. The third concerns the relationship of the words to the non-verbal aspects of the communication, e.g. gestures and facial expressions.

Touch

Fredrickson (1999) also relates to the importance of task-oriented touch during any interaction. Routasalo (1999) describes two types of touch: physical and therapeutic. It may be suggested that there is a very definite purpose to therapeutic touch, which is aimed at the well-being of the patient. Touch must be used with care. Davidhizar and Giger (1997) report that most health-care professionals believe in the value of touch in caring relationships. When supporting a relative of a patient who is dying it may be appropriate to hold that person's hand. However, this is not true for every health-care professional and some patients may not see touch as appropriate or desirable. Shaking hands is a good method of introducing yourself to the patient, but not every patient likes to shake hands. It is therefore important that a professional is aware of the indications within a situation (such as the reaction of the patient to a handshake), which can help to decide whether touch should be used.

Individual personalities

Other non-verbal aspects of communication can play a part within the health professional–patient relationship. According to Sand (2003), these include factors relevant to the personality of the nurse, and the motivation and the professional conduct of the nurse are also important. Personality will affect the methods used to cope with stress and anxiety and these will reflect on the nurse–patient relationship. An example is the student nurse's facial responses to a patient's request, when he or she is busy (Bond 1986). This will affect the rapport that is established between the health professional and the patient.

This section of the chapter has suggested that the issues involved within non-verbal communication are both diverse and many. The difference between communication and effective communication can be apparent in the way non-verbal and active listening skills are used. The effective use of these non-verbal communication skills can have a very positive effect on the patient's care.

The world of interpersonal skills

Communication suggests conveying a message from one individual to another. The 'personal' part of the word 'interpersonal' is suggestive of an issue specific to an individual. Concepts which are inherent to interpersonal skills include:

• self-awareness
• assertiveness
• the ability to use empathy.

Events of an interpersonal nature therefore suggest that the communication involved is of a much more individualistic nature between the parties and may relate to issues that are very personal to both.

The importance of communication within interpersonal relationships is reflected by the individual's desire to pass on or receive knowledge. To develop an interpersonal understanding with another person means that such knowledge acquisition can take place more effectively. Ellis (1992) discusses how some people are very flexible in their approach to different communication styles. They have an ability to talk very objectively and straightforwardly about an issue that, in practice, they may feel very deeply about and have very personal views on. These people have a high level of self-awareness and can use their own interpersonal skills to bring out a far greater and more effective interaction with the other person. An example is being able to appear motivated and content even when the day has not gone well. Patients will often respond well to the health professional who can make patients laugh even when they themselves do not feel like doing so. Niven (1989) cites the idea proposed by Luft and Ingham (1955), called the Johari window. The basis of the idea is that there are four aspects of the self:

- The open self
- The blind self
- The hidden self
- The unknown self.

Table 4.1 describes what each aspect of the self means in practice.

Table 4.1 Aspects of the self

Open self	Blind self
Details of issues in a conversation are known to us and known to others	Details of issues in a conversation are unknown to us but known to others
Hidden self	Unknown self
Details of issues in a conversation are known to us but unknown to others (i.e. they are hidden)	Details of issues that are important in a conversation are unknown to us as well as to others

An example of the importance of the concept of the Johari window when considering the implications of interpersonal skills for a student nurse is given below.

Open self

A student nurse who visits a patient at home and takes his temperature may indicate in discussions that she is upset that the patient's temperature is high. The student nurse also states that this is because of the patient's current chest infection. The patient knows that the student is aware of the chest infection from previous discussions with the student, but is now fully aware of how the student feels about his condition.

Blind self

In this example, the student nurse who takes a patient's temperature is unaware of the reasons why she is doing so. The patient is fully aware of the implications if his temperature is high (i.e. that he will still have the chest infection and that he may be admitted to hospital). The conversation between the two people would reflect this and it could be that the patient does not wish to reveal the implications of the high temperature to the student nurse for fear of the consequences of doing so.

Hidden self

Alternatively, the student nurse may know that the high temperature indicates that the patient's chest infection is getting worse and that this means hospitalization. However, she does not relay this fact to the patient, preferring to speak to a more experienced nurse back at the health clinic first. Therefore, for the time being the patient would remain ill-informed about his condition.

Unknown self

Both the student nurse and the patient are unaware of why the patient's temperature is being taken other than the fact that the doctor has requested it. It may be that the doctor suspects a condition but has not made his or her suspicions known to either the student nurse or the patient.

Being skilled in interpersonal relationships will increase the amount of self-disclosure so that the patient knows more about the health-care practitioner, and allowing the patient to make more effective decisions. If the student is able to demonstrate his or her 'open self', in the example above, the patient is likely to feel that the student nurse is genuinely concerned about his or her condition and will therefore negotiate an appropriate course of action with the student nurse. The situation in which care is being given to the patient by the student nurse has, therefore, been improved. The process also allows the student concerned to get an insight into his or her own feelings from the conversation, as the patient is likely to provide a response to how the student feels.

The ability to become self-aware helps the nurse to become assertive by allowing him or her to decide how to increase the level of self-disclosure in a quick, safe and effective way. The student nurse who gives the patient confident advice, based on what the district nurse has informed him or her, and requests that he or she carry out the procedure in a certain way is being assertive in his or her manner. Being assertive is not being aggressive, manipulative or submissive (Bond 1986). The student nurse who becomes angry because the patient is not following the district nurse's instructions can easily appear aggressive. The student nurse who persists in giving the patient false information to achieve hidden agendas can easily become manipulative and one who offers rewards in order to be able to visit the patient (e.g. offering to collect the patient's prescription on the way to the patient's house) can become submissive. Effective interpersonal skills rely on the student nurse being honest, open and having a level of confidence in dealing with the patient.

The effective use of self-disclosure and assertiveness skills can assist in enabling the health professional to empathize effectively with the patient. Ellis (1992) describes empathy as having a 'with you' quality about it that enables the student nurse to go beyond intellectual understanding or showing sympathy. Empathy does not require a student nurse to give the patient a firm answer to an emotional question when that is not possible or even desirable. The patient's feelings can be accepted without any judgements being applied to them by the health professional. This may well enable the patient to explore his or her own feelings while the student nurse is there. The student nurse is prepared to listen actively and to give the patient commitment and time during this process.

Becoming or being involved in situations that demand empathy can allow a unique insight into the individual world of a patient. Such events require interpersonal skills (incorporating verbal and non-verbal communication skills) to be used effectively. When this happens the professional relationship becomes enhanced as both the health professional's and the patient's knowledge and understanding grow in partnership.

The use and development of communication and interpersonal skills in the practice setting

So far, some of the components of communication and interpersonal skills have been examined, but the question now arises of how the novice practitioner develops and enhances these skills in the practice setting. This process starts by making an assumption that learning about such skills will be part of a professional development process. Having mastered basic concepts in communication and interpersonal qualities, the nurse will be in a position to recognize issues that hinder their ability to be effective in using those skills. A number of issues are given below and the individual needs to be particularly careful to avoid engaging in such communicative behaviours (adapted from Robertson and O'Kell 1992):

• mumbling
• using multiple questions at once
• interrupting
• distracting

- asking inappropriate questions
- arguing
- passing judgement
- jumping to conclusions
- devaluing the person
- using harsh language
- being bored or impatient.

Texts have been written to support the process of development; examples include Maxim and Bryan (1995) and work by Robertson and O'Kell (1992). The latter suggest ideas for interacting with visually and hearing-impaired patients. Examples are given in Table 4.2.

Table 4.2 How to interact with visually and hearing-impaired patients

Visual impairment	Hearing impairment
Identify yourself	Speak loudly but do not shout
Explain clearly	Maintain eye contact
Ask for feedback	Eliminate unnecessary noise
Offer spectacles	Ensure that hearing aid is on
Use touch where appropriate	Face person who lipreads

Maxim and Bryan (1995) consider how illness affects the patient's ability to communicate and the implications that this process has for the health professional. They suggest that some patients may become over-cheerful whereas others become very quiet and withdrawn. A patient may be very embarrassed about having to request assistance to help them bathe. Some patients may even become angry or abusive. Clear explanations (given calmly and slowly) on the part of the health professional are therefore important to indicate what his or her intentions are in relation to any nursing procedure about to be carried out in negotiation with the patient. Some patients may have specific illnesses; these could include patients who have had a cerebrovascular accident (stroke) or those who may have a language disorder. Maxim and Bryan (1995) make the following recommendations in communicating with these patients:

- Slow down.
- Remove distractions.
- Break any speech into stages, e.g.:
  'It's getting cold, isn't it?'
  'Are you cold?'
  'Do you want a blanket?'
- Maintain eye contact with the person while he or she struggles to speak.
- Look interested.
- Give the person time to speak.

- Commiserate with the person if he or she becomes upset.
- Use normal voice and expression.
- Ask the person's opinion.
- Use gesture.
- Do not expect the person to speak for too long. Remember that speaking may be an effort.

Communication and interpersonal skills: the process of reflection

Reflection has been suggested as a means of integrating the 'person of the nurse' with the 'person of the patient' (Boykin and Schoenhofer 1993). This allows individuals to learn directly from interactions with patients on a daily basis. For the health professional to learn from a relevant situation, aspects of the event need to be examined (in this case involving communication or interpersonal skills). Gibbs (1988) has offered a method in which the process can be undertaken, and a method of learning from it, through a series of questions. There are six questions in the framework, which allows the health professional constantly to learn from the experience. Gibbs' framework or cycle is given in Figure 4.1.

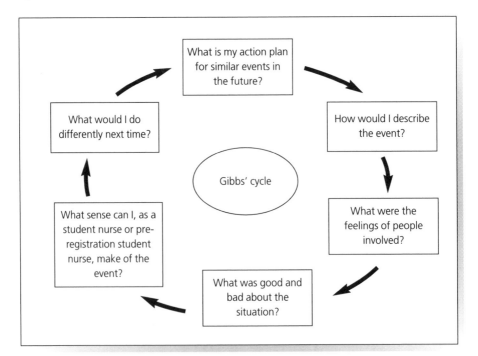

Figure 4.1
Gibbs' cycle
(Gibbs 1988).

Each question within Gibbs' cycle is examined and an example worked through to illustrate how the reflection can proceed effectively.

Description of the event

For the student nurse to reflect on a situation effectively, he or she must be very clear about the parts of the situation that make up the event.

The feelings of the people involved

The feelings of each person within the event need to be considered. The language of 'feelings' is used. The student nurse may, for example, be very *worried* about the patient's ability to keep him- or herself warm. He or she may also have *felt* that the patient might be *disgruntled* should the nurse not respond to his or her call for assistance. The student nurse may therefore be *concerned* about the patient's health

What was good and bad about the situation?

The student nurse must decide what was good and bad about the event. The positive aspects of a situation may suggest that the student nurse feels able to listen and respond to the patient's call for assistance, suggesting that the health professional and patient had a good rapport with each other. Morrison and Burnard (1991) discuss how important honesty is in the effective use of interpersonal skills.

What sense can I make of the event?

This reflective process requires that the student nurse take a look at why he or she conducted the interaction in this way. Morrison and Burnard (1991) also state that trust is a requirement for caring, and they suggest that health professionals should allow patients the opportunity to trust themselves. The responsibility for the patient in heating his or her own home is his or hers. Although a health professional can give support within the task, he or she must never allow personal values to result in the patient being deceived into believing the wrong reasons for an action undertaken by that health professional.

What would I do differently next time?

So that health professionals can decide what action needs to be taken to enhance learning, it is important that they consider how they may have reacted differently in the situation. The essence of this reflection suggests that student nurses need to learn to be honest with patients. Trusting patients may require health professionals to understand that patients may decide to take actions that student nurses would perhaps rather they did not take. Student nurses need to develop confidence in dealing with situations where this occurs so that they can use the appropriate communication and interpersonal skills next time.

What is my action plan for similar events in the future?

So that student nurses can be more open and honest in situations such as this, they may need to learn skills such as assertiveness. Through their employers it may be possible to access such a course; if not, such courses are often open to the public through education programmes offered in colleges of further education.

The content of reflective practice pertaining to communication and interpersonal skills

The suggestion has already been made that the particular issues upon which an individual's reflective practice should be based depend on the health professional's experience. This ensures not only that reflection is personal, but also that the reflector is able to develop as a result of the reflection. For the nurse who has not actively reflected before (by using a recognized reflective process such as Gibbs' cycle), the identification of a suitable topic related to communication or interpersonal skills may prove difficult. Literature such as the works of Porritt (1990) can offer ideas and it is possible to put some of those in the context of what has been discussed so far.

The resulting ideas have been put in the form of questions, which individuals may wish to ask themselves (Table 4.3).

Table 4.3 Self-assessment questions

Developing your verbal communication	Do you reflect on your tone of voice when you speak? Do you use open and closed questions appropriately?
Developing your non-verbal communication and listening skills	Do you use your body in a way that is consistent with what you are saying? Do you always demonstrate that you are maintaining attention while a patient is talking to you? Do you reflect back on what someone is telling you?
Developing your interpersonal skills	Do you use self-disclosure effectively? Can you be assertive without being aggressive, manipulative or submissive? Can you use empathy effectively?
Developing your communication and interpersonal skills	Can you recognize barriers that prevent you from communicating effectively? Can you communicate with patients who have visual or hearing impediments? Are you aware of any specific aspects of communication or interpersonal skills that may be relevant to a patient for whom you care (e.g. those relevant to a patient with a stroke may be pertinent if you care for that sort of patient)?

Cont.

Table 4.3 *Cont.*

Reflection	Are you ready to begin to work through a process of reflection? Can you be self-critical? Can you evaluate aspects of your own performance? Are you adaptable and able to incorporate things that you learn into your future practice?

Conclusion

This chapter has taken the reader on a journey, which started with very concrete information on the subject of communication. It quickly travelled into more diverse concepts in which the whole idea of good interpersonal skills was offered as a basis for effective patient care. However, in order to participate in this journey it should now be evident that the reader has to believe four things. First, that communication and interpersonal skills can be learned. Second, that the pupil can make great strides to learn these skills him- or herself (although not suggesting that this would be any substitute for a programme of learning). Third, that the practice setting combined with reflective practice enables the reader to develop and enhance such skills in their interactions with patients. Finally, those interpersonal skills that can appear to matter most are the most fundamental of all, such as forming a rapport with your patient and having the ability to listen to him or her in a way that is appreciated by the person and even fellow health-care team members.

People are discovering new facts about communication and interpersonal skills every day and reflection can be part of that process. Through reflection we can explore the world of communication and interpersonal skills for ourselves. Today we may undertake the reflective process as a student nurse and the day after as part of our life-long learning process. The result is that our understanding of issues such as verbal and non-verbal skills, listening, assertiveness and empathy can increase after each event that we choose to reflect upon. This chapter has encouraged readers to take that journey of reflection and to explore the exciting world of communication and interpersonal skills for themselves.

References

Bond, M. (1986) Stress and Self-awareness: A guide for nurses. Oxford: Heinemann Nursing.

Boyd, E. and Fales, A. (1983) Reflecting learning: Key to learning from experience. Journal of Humanistic Psychology 23: 99–117.

Boykin, A. and Schoenhofer, S. (1993) Nursing as Caring: A model for transforming practice. New York: National League for Nursing Press.

Caris-Verhallen, W., Kerkstra, A. and Bensing Jozien, M. (1999) Non-verbal behaviour in nurse–elderly patient communication. Journal of Advanced Nursing 29: 808–818.

Davidhizar, R. and Giger, J. (1997) When touch is not the best approach. Journal of Clinical Nursing 6: 203–206.

Ellis, R. (1992) The nurse as communicator. In: Kenworthy, N., Snowley, G. and Gilling, C. (eds), Common Foundation Studies in Nursing. Edinburgh: Churchill Livingstone.

Fredrickson, L. (1999) Modes of relating in a caring conversation: a research synthesis on presence, touch and listening. Journal of Advanced Nursing 30: 1167–1176.

Gibbs, G. (1988) Learning by Doing: A guide to teaching and learning methods. Oxford: Further Education Unit, Oxford Polytechnic.

Kimura, D. and Seal, B. (2003) Sex differences in recall of real or nonsense words. Psychological Reports 93: 263–264.

Luft, J. and Ingham, H. (1955) The Johari Window: A graphic model for interpersonal relationships. University of California, Western Training Laboratory in Group Development. Cited in Niven (1989).

Maxim, J. and Bryan, K. (1995) Talking and listening. In: Darby, S. and Benson, S. (eds), Community Care Assistants and Support Workers. London: Hawker Publications.

Morrison, P. and Burnard, P. (1991) Caring and Communicating. Basingstoke: Macmillan Press.

Niven, N. (1989) Health Psychology. Edinburgh: Churchill Livingstone.

Porritt, L. (1990) Interaction Strategies. Melbourne: Churchill Livingstone.

Robertson, B. and O'Kell, S. (1992) Health and Social Care Support Workers: 10 step by step support modules, 2nd edn. Bristol: First Class Books.

Rodriguez-Aranda, C. (2003) Reduced writing and reading speed and age-related changes in verbal fluency tasks. The Clinical Psychologist 17: 203–215.

Routasalo, P. (1999) Physical touch in nursing studies: a literature review. Journal of Advanced Nursing 30: 843–850.

Sand, A. (2003) Nurses' personalities, nursing-related qualities and work satisfaction: a 10 year perspective. Journal of Clinical Nursing 6: 177–187.

Shakespeare, P. (2003) Nurse's bodywork: is there a body of work? Nursing Inquiry 10(1): 47–56.

Siditis, D. (2004) When novel sentences spoken or heard for the first time in the history of the universe are not enough: toward a dual-process model of language. International Journal of Language and Communication Disorders 39: 1–44.

CHAPTER 5

Breathing and respiration

CHRISTINE GAULT

Breathing is essential for life; it occurs so that the bloodstream can transport oxygen to cells of the body. Jenkins (2003) points out that as a rule breathing is an independent activity occurring immediately after birth. Roper et al. (2000) state that breathing can be effortless and people are not usually consciously aware of this activity of living, until certain abnormal conditions force the individual to become consciously aware of it.

Epstein et al. (1997) suggest that diseases associated with the respiratory tract account for the highest number of general practitioner consultations. The effects of respiratory tract disease impinge on all activities of living and the disease is also responsible for the highest number of days lost from work.

To care effectively for patients who have diseases of the respiratory tract the nurse will need to understand the role that the respiratory tract plays in the metabolism of the cells of the body (Cutler and Murch 2003). The nurse's role in assessing a patient with a respiratory disease is outlined in this chapter. The complexities of breathing are only briefly addressed here and the reader is advised to refer to other texts on the subject in order to understand fully the physiological principles and resulting nursing care.

Structure and function of the respiratory tract

The respiratory tract extends from the nose to the alveoli of the lungs. The lungs and respiratory passages are shown in Figure 5.1.

Respiration

One of the key requirements of the cells in the human body is to receive oxygen (O_2). The bloodstream delivers O_2, protein, fats and glucose; these products enable the body to produce energy (known as catabolism). Carbon dioxide (CO_2), a poison in high concentrations, produced by the cells along with water (H_2O – a process known as metabolism), is excreted through the process of respiration which occurs via the lungs. Without this process humans would die.

Figure 5.1
Aspects of the
respiratory system
and related
structures.

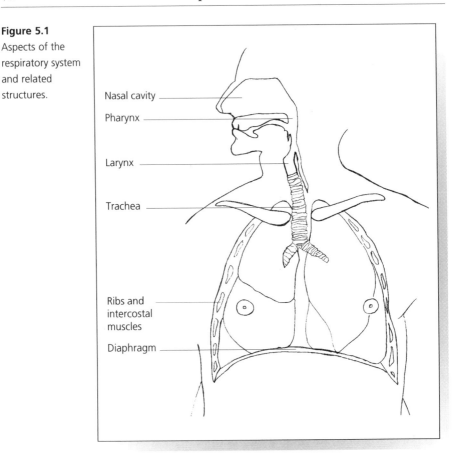

Nasal cavity

Pharynx

Larynx

Trachea

Ribs and
intercostal
muscles

Diaphragm

Control of breathing

Regulation of respiration is complex and is essentially controlled by the brain in response to two factors: neural and chemical (Sadik and Elliott 2002). Normal breathing is known as eupnoea (Cutler and Murch 2003).

Neural control

The respiratory centre is situated in the medulla oblongata in the brain. Along with the pons varolii it produces nervous impulses that influence breathing (Martini 2001). During inhalation, when tension is reached on the walls of the bronchi, the vagus nerve (tenth cranial nerve) passes an impulse to the bronchi. The respiratory centre sends nerve impulses to the diaphragm and intercostal muscles to relax, and expiration occurs; this causes the thoracic cage to enlarge. These actions are involuntary and as such occur unconsciously. Voluntary actions are activities over which we have some degree of control; they include coughing or sneezing when stimulated by irritating substances.

Chemical control

Control of respiration by chemical stimulation is achieved by the actions of a specialized group of cells known as chemoreceptors, which are situated in the walls of the aorta and the carotid arteries. In addition, the carotid sinus of the carotid artery is sensitive to an excess of CO_2 and a deficiency of O_2. The resultant changes associated with either high or low levels of O_2 or CO_2 (partial pressures) can send nerve impulses to the respiratory centre to alter the rate and depth of breathing (Hogston and Simpson 2002).

The bronchi

Air passes into the lungs from the trachea and bronchi. Initially air is filtered, saturated with water vapour and warmed by the nose. It then passes through the pharynx and larynx and down into the trachea and bronchi (Figure 5.2).

There are two bronchi; they start at the bifurcation of the trachea and each bronchus leads to a lung, either right or left (Whittaker 2004). The right bronchus is more vertical and shorter than the left; the left bronchus is

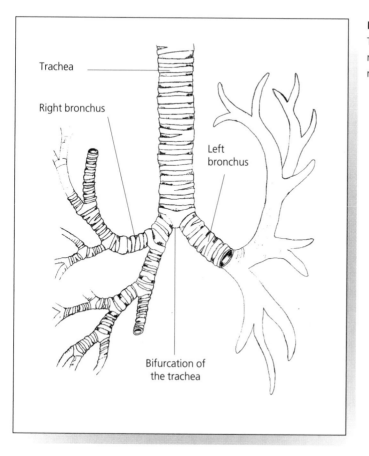

Figure 5.2
The main, left and right bronchi (lungs removed).

Trachea

Right bronchus

Left bronchus

Bifurcation of the trachea

slightly smaller and narrower than the right as a result of the position of the heart within the mediastinum. Each of the bronchi divides into branches corresponding to each of the lobes of the lung.

Lining of the respiratory system

The trachea is lined with small cells called columnar epithelial cells. These cells have small hair-like projections called cilia, which are covered with mucus (produced by the bronchial glands); they will trap foreign or dirt particles, which if causing irritation can usually be coughed up by the individual.

The diaphragm

This muscle is shaped like a dome that separates the thorax from the abdomen. This sheet of muscle fibres connects to fibrous tissue known as the central tendon. Phrenic nerves on either side of the diaphragm cause the diaphragm to contract. The respiratory centre, situated in the brain (the medulla oblongata), controls this action.

Accessory muscles

Anterior to the wall of the chest is the pectoralis major muscle, around the lateral wall is the serratus anterior muscle and the sternomastoid muscle passes from the back of the skull to the clavicle. Although the main function of these muscles is for movement of the head, arms and scapulae, they may also assist when breathing becomes difficult. This group of muscles helps respiration by moving the ribcage (Sadik and Elliott 2002).

The lungs

There are two lungs, and it should be noted that the right lung has three lobes – upper, middle and lower lobe – whereas the left lung is made up of two lobes – upper and lower lobe. Both lungs are conical in shape, with the base on the diaphragm and the apex reaching up towards the clavicle (Figure 5.3).

Surrounding each lung is the pleura, which is a continuous membrane that folds back on itself. At the root of the lung is the parietal pleura covering the interior of the chest, the mediastinum and the diaphragm. The inner layer is the visceral pleura, which covers the lungs; between both these layers is a potential space – the pleural space.

The alveoli

The alveoli are the terminal ends of the bronchioles (Figure 5.4). It is here that gaseous exchange takes place.

These minute terminal bronchioles form tiny air passages known as alveolar ducts, which open into alveolar sacs (Whittaker 2004). The walls of

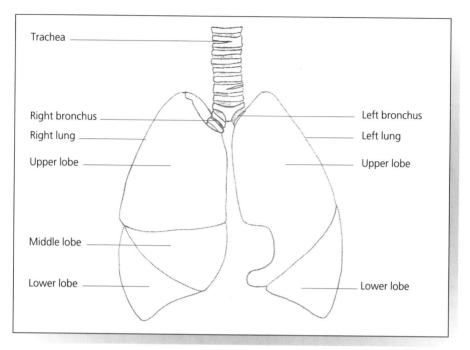

Figure 5.3
The lungs: right lung with three lobes and left lung with two lobes (note the heart space).

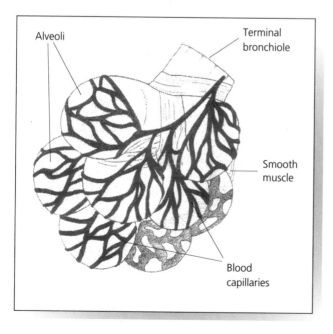

Figure 5.4
The alveoli, terminal bronchiole and capillary network.

the alveoli are single-thickness, squamous epithelial cells (Martini 2001). Externally, the alveoli are surrounded by a very thin pulmonary capillary network. There are millions of alveoli providing a large surface area which is greatly increased by the alveolar walls. Air and blood are separated by two layers of cells and a layer of moisture: the alveolus wall and the capillary wall; together they form the respiratory membrane. On one side of this membrane there are gases and on the other side there is a fast flowing bloodstream enabling gases to move rapidly between air and blood. Simple diffusion allows gas exchange to occur. Deoxygenated blood enters the capillary network via the pulmonary artery and as this occurs (by simple diffusion) oxygenated blood leaves the network entering the pulmonary veins. There are millions of gas-filled alveoli in the lungs, which allow for massive amounts of gas to be exchanged (Marieb 2004).

Assessment of respiration

Respiratory assessment involves observation of the patient, collecting information, including the measurement of respiratory function, and physical examination. The nurse will need to speak to the patient to obtain a history; however, caution must be used because the patient may be so short of breath that encouraging him or her to speak may be detrimental to his or her health. Secondary data (data collected from a variety of sources other than the patient) may have to suffice if the nurse is unable to gain primary data (data given to the nurse by the patient). Data may be given to the nurse by other health-care professionals or significant others, or taken from the patient's nursing/medical notes. Chapter 2 describes the assessment process generally; this section concentrates on how to assess the patient's respiratory needs, confidently and competently, in order to gain insight into this complex activity of living.

Breathing should normally be effortless. Breathlessness may be accompanied by the use of the accessory muscles, so distress may be visual. The nurse can learn much from the patient by accurate observation. The rate, depth and rhythm must be noted, and the nurse should observe the chest wall to see whether it moves equally on both sides. The skill of listening is also required and the nurse must be alert to any noises that are made during inspiration and expiration.

Jenkins (2003) makes it clear that to assess breathing effectively the nurse must give due consideration to aspects of Roper et al.'s (1996) model of nursing:

- Lifespan: consider effect of age on breathing
- Dependency: linked to lifespan and ill-health
- Independence: linked to health
- Factors affecting breathing:
  - *biological:*
    - degree of physical activity

- body's physiological responses to stressors
- intact respiratory system to enable effective internal and external respiration
- intact circulatory system and nervous system
- noted by observation of normal breathing
- note any abnormal breathing, i.e. wheeze, sputum production
- *psychological:* effect of emotional state on breathing, i.e. anxiety, panic, fear
- *sociocultural:* expectoration of sputum and coughing habits
- *environmental:*
  - exposure to micro-organisms
  - exposure to air pollutants at home or at work
- *politicoeconomic:* mechanisms to limit smoking-related diseases and air pollutant diseases.

Measuring respiratory rate, depth and rhythm

When assessing the patient's respiratory status the nurse must assess the rate, depth and pattern of respiration (rhythm). The normal resting respiratory rate in the adult is 12-16 breaths/minute, with expiration taking nearly twice as long as inspiration (Grandis et al. 2003).

Respiratory assessment is carried out by the nurse to determine a baseline observation, which allows the nurse to make a comparison at a later date. The nurse may also use respiratory assessment to evaluate how the patient has responded to medications or treatments that have been given for a respiratory disease.

The nurse must be aware that respiratory rate, depth and rhythm can be altered by a patient who is aware that the nurse is measuring this activity. The nurse should attempt to assess the patient's respiratory status without his or her knowledge.

Respiratory rate is the number of inspirations and expirations that the patient makes in one minute while at rest. It is therefore important that the respiratory rate is not assessed after the patient has undergone any form of exercise because an incorrect finding may be recorded.

Procedure for assessing the patient's respiratory status

- Explain the procedure to the patient, but do not inform him or her when you will be undertaking the activity.
- A more accurate assessment of respiratory rate, depth and rhythm will occur if the nurse does not alert the patient to the fact that he or she is observing this activity. Some nurses may pretend to be taking the radial pulse when in fact they are counting and observing respiratory function.
- The nurse will need a watch with a second hand.
- The nurse observes movement of the chest wall and counts the

respirations for 60 seconds (do not be tempted to do this for 30 seconds and double your findings because this could be detrimental to your patient's health).
• Observe the rhythm and depth of respiratory effort. Depth of respiration is best assessed by observing the amount of movement made by the chest wall. The measurement of depth will relate to the amount of air being moved into and out of the lungs.

The nurse must document the observations in the patient's nursing notes and report any respiratory abnormalities. He or she may need to alter or adjust the frequency of observation as the patient's condition dictates. Respiratory effort can be categorized as:

• Rapid, shallow breathing – in excess of 20 breaths/minute is termed 'tachypnoea' and may be the result of an increase in activity, anxiety, fear, pain or pyrexia. This can be caused by the body's response to extra demands being made on it – a need for extra oxygen.
• A decrease in respiration to less than 12 breaths/minute is known as bradypnoea and may be caused by the effects of strong medications such as opiates (i.e. morphine), sleep, head injury, brain lesion or hypothermia. This type of breathing is slow but regular.
• Apnoea occurs when the patient fails to breathe for at least 10 seconds. Apnoea may precede or occur immediately after cardiac/respiratory arrest.
• Cheyne–Stokes breathing is characterized by a waxing and waning of respiratory depth over a minute or more. Respiratory depth may be deep and may become almost absent. This type of respiratory effort is often seen in patients who are terminally ill and may occur immediately before death.

Respiratory sounds

In some instances when respiratory disease is present the patient may make audible respiratory sounds; in 'normal' respiration no sound is heard. The sounds made may indicate or alert the nurse to specific type of illness so she or he must be aware of these sounds and their possible meanings. Table 5.1 outlines the names given to particular sounds that the patient may make when respiratory disease is present.

Assessment of the patient with a respiratory disease will include observation of the skin for signs of cyanosis. When tissue oxygenation is low or high there may be some particular signs that will alert the nurse to this. When cyanosis (a bluish or purplish discoloration of the skin or mucous membranes) is present, this indicates a reduction in haemoglobin in the blood. Central cyanosis (a bluish tinge to the mucous membranes of the mouth – buccal mucosa, the lips and conjunctivae) indicates serious lung

Table 5.1 Respiratory sounds and their potential meanings

Name of sound	Potential meaning
Wheeze	Wheeze is a high-pitched whistling sound. It can occur in inspiration and expiration but is often loudest in expiration. It implies narrowing of the lower airway and is common in asthma (Hogston and Simpson 2002)
Stridor	A harsh sound heard on inspiration and expiration can indicate obstruction of the larynx (Epstein et al. 1997)
Snoring	Usually occurs during sleep and may indicate an obstruction of the airway. The obstruction may be nasal, oropharyngeal or laryngeal. Sleep apnoea may occur if snoring is severe and can lead to hypoxic episodes (Epstein et al. 1997)
Râles and crepitations	Heard when a stethoscope is placed on the chest wall and may indicate pulmonary oedema (Sadik and Elliott 2002)

and/or heart disease or any disease that prevents adequate oxygenation of the blood (Street 2003). Peripheral cyanosis involves the extremities, i.e. the hands and feet, although the tongue (as opposed to central cyanosis) remains a healthy pink colour.

Observation of cough and sputum

Cough

The characteristics of the cough, together with other symptoms, may give an indication of the cause. Cough is a result of irritation to the cough receptors in the pharynx, larynx and bronchi. The nurse should note the presence, frequency, depth, nature and sound of the cough (Jenkins 2003). Furthermore, the nurse should note whether the cough has any effect on the patient's ability to carry out the activities of living, i.e. to communicate or sleep.

According to Johnson et al. (2000), cough may be caused by:

- infection
- physical and chemical stimuli
- circulatory problems
- cancer
- habit.

The cough may be productive, i.e. sputum is expectorated when the patient coughs, or non-productive or dry – when little or no sputum is produced.

Sputum

It is usual for an adult to produce approximately 100 ml sputum/day (Walsh 2002). Law (2000) states that there are many types of sputum and the amount produced can vary from 100 to 500 ml/day. The amount of sputum produced when the respiratory tract is irritated or inflamed will increase. Patients may refer to sputum as phlegm; if this is the case the nurse must use this word when questioning the patient.

The nurse needs, from time to time, to observe, note and report the type of sputum the patient is producing. The following should be noted and documented in the patient's nursing notes:

* quantity
* consistency
* colour
* odour.

The clinical features of sputum are as follows (Epstein et al. 1997, Law 2000).

* White or grey:
    - smoking
    - chronic bronchitis
    - asthma
* Yellow or green:
    - acute bronchitis
    - asthma
    - bronchiectasis
    - cystic fibrosis
* Frothy, blood stained:
    - pulmonary oedema
* Haemoptysis (bleeding into the lungs)
    - bright red secretions and froth may indicate that the patient has tuberculosis, carcinoma of the lung, trauma or pulmonary embolism.

To determine the cause of sputum production and to aid with diagnosis the nurse must ask the patient specific questions. The following are some useful questions to ask:

* What colour is the sputum (phlegm)?
* How often are you coughing it up?
* How much do you cough up?
* Do you have difficulty coughing it up?
* Do you use anything from the doctor or the chemist's to help you with the sputum (phlegm)?

Although it is important to assess the type of sputum the patient produces and to ask pertinent questions such as those above, the nurse may need to obtain a sputum specimen in order to confirm or to make an accurate diagnosis.

Procedure for collecting a sputum specimen

The nurse is advised to adhere to local policy and procedure for collecting a sputum specimen for analysis. Outlined below are some points that should be considered when collecting a sputum specimen:

Equipment needed for the collection of sputum specimen

- Sterile, leak-proof container
- Specimen bag and request form with the laboratory tests required noted on it.

The procedure

- Explain carefully in a way that the patient will understand why the specimen is needed. Ensure privacy.
- If the patient is to be commenced on prescribed antibacterial medication, the nurse should endeavour to collect the sputum before the course of antibiotics is started.
- Before starting the collection of sputum, ask the patient to rinse the mouth with water because this will remove oral plaque and secretions that may contaminate the specimen.
- Point out that the patient needs to provide a sputum specimen, not a specimen of saliva or mucus from the postnasal space.
- Provide the patient with a sterile sputum pot for collection of the specimen if she or he is able to do this independently with tissues at hand.
- Explain that contamination of the inside of the pot by her or his fingers should be avoided because this will interfere with an accurate analysis of sputum from the lung and may impede diagnosis and subsequent treatment.
- Encourage the patient to breathe deeply to stimulate coughing expectoration and to loosen secretions.
- If the patient is experiencing difficulty expectorating, the nurse may assist by providing a eucalyptus inhalation (Sadik and Elliott 2002).
- In some cases the nurse may need to instigate, with the assistance of the physiotherapist, postural drainage to encourage the removal of secretions.
- The specimen should be refrigerated until processing takes place.
- Document your actions and also record in the nursing notes the colour, smell and consistency of the sputum.

A sputum specimen may be easier to obtain from the patient if collected early in the morning. As the patient has been sleeping through the night and the respiratory rate is slower and the depth of breathing shallower, there may be more of a chance for secretions to have accumulated in the lung (Daniels 2002).

Other methods of assessing respiratory function

Pulse oximetry (Figure 5.5)

Pulse oximetry enables the nurse to measure the O_2 saturation of haemoglobin; this is a non-invasive technique and is represented by the following notation - SaO_2. The oximeter probe is attached to the finger, toe or ear lobe. The normal level is 95–99% (Nicol et al. 2000); if the SaO_2 falls below 85% the reading becomes less reliable (Bassett and Makin 2000). It is important to note that the oximeter can take up to 30 seconds to detect a fall in O_2 concentration, which could be a critical time for instigating treatment or therapy. To obtain an accurate reading the nurse should ensure that:

- the probe has been positioned correctly, ensuring a good flow of blood to the area
- there is no nail varnish on the finger or toe nails
- there is no direct overhead light
- the patient is not shivering
- there is no mechanical movement of the probe.

The nurse must ensure that he or she has documented in the nursing notes the SaO_2 and whether the patient is receiving O_2 therapy. Any changes or abnormalities must be reported immediately

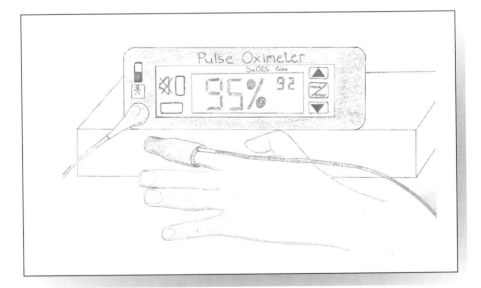

Figure 5.5
The pulse oximeter and
sensor attached.

Peak expiratory flow rate

The peak expiratory flow rate (PEFR) allows the nurse to note objectively how much air the patient can empty from his or her lungs in litres per minute; it measures the individual's ability to exhale (Baillie et al. 2001). It is important that the nurse understands how to measure and record the PEFR because it is one of the most commonly used methods to assess the patient's respiratory status.

The PEFR is most often recorded to assess and monitor the effects of treatment. Woolons (1995) notes that patients with asthma often experience problems with lung capacity and variable obstruction of the airways. As a result, it is often (but not exclusively) the patient with asthma for whom the nurse will use the PEFR measurement. It is recommended that a PEFR be performed before and after treatment, such as a nebulizer or inhaler, has been given to assess the effectiveness and efficacy of the medications. In this case, the PEFR should be recorded approximately 20 minutes after the medication has been given (Nicol et al. 2000).

The procedure for measuring PEFR

Equipment needed

- Chart to record measurement
- Peak flowmeter
- Disposable mouthpiece.

Procedure

- Explain the reason for the procedure and how you intend to carry it out.
- PEFR is best measured if the patient is standing up. If the patient is unable to do this then he or she should be sitting in a chair or sitting upright in bed.
- Attach disposable mouthpiece.
- Set the peak flowmeter at zero.
- Instruct the patient to inhale deeply, place the lips around the mouthpiece and, holding the meter horizontally, exhale forcibly.
- Note the measurement.
- Repeat twice.
- Record the highest of the three measurements. The dial attached to the peak flowmeter should be returned to the lowest setting in between each attempt.

The procedure may bring about coughing or wheezing. If this is the case the nurse should ask the patient to attempt the procedure only once and this should be noted on the chart.

Aerosols and nebulizers

Aerosolization and nebulization are two methods of drug administration that allow the inhalation of a variety of drugs with the aim of localized therapeutic effect (Mallett and Dougherty 2000). The most common types of drugs that are used via inhalation in the UK are bronchodilators and steroids (Baillie et al. 2001).

Aerosols

Over 90% of people with asthma take the medications that they require by inhalation. There are a variety of inhaler devices available and the most common type is the metered dose inhaler. The patient needs a great deal of skill and the ability to coordinate for effective administration. The nurse has an educational role to play in teaching the patient or carer how to administer the inhaler correctly in order to ensure that the correct dose is delivered to the patient. The Asthma Training Centre (1997) estimates that one in five people do not use their inhaler correctly.

The main principles for using an aerosol

- Ensure that the medication (the inhaler) is the correct medication prescribed for the patient.
- Remove the cover of the inhaler and shake the inhaler.
- Ask the patient to breathe out gently but not fully.
- When the patient's head is tilted slightly backwards, place the mouthpiece between the lips and ask the patient to breathe in as deeply as possible; activate the inhaler at the start of inspiration.
- Remove the inhaler from between the lips.
- The patient holds his or her breath for 10 seconds and then breathes out slowly.
- Repeat the procedure if necessary and as prescribed.
- The drug should be signed for on the drug administration sheet in the normal and accepted manner. The nurse must record the effect of the medication in the patient's notes.

Nebulizers

A nebulizer is attached to a flow of air or O_2 and converts a solution of the prescribed drug (with 2–3 ml physiological [0.9%] saline) into an aerosol for inhalation. Nebulizer therapy is usually administered three to four times a day and the administration of the nebulizer must be consistent with local policy and procedure.

Some common respiratory diseases

Asthma

Asthma is a chronic inflammatory condition of the airways. The term 'asthma' is derived from the Greek word meaning 'panting' (Bassett and Makin 2000). The cause of this disease is still not completely understood

(Brewin 1997). It is characterized by spasm of the bronchial muscles and oedema of the bronchial mucosa, resulting in recurrent attacks of wheezing, vocally, during expiration. Narrowing of the airways occurs as a response to stimuli such as infection, allergy or unknown cause. Bronchoconstriction occurs and breathing becomes difficult (dyspnoea) and laboured. McEwing et al. (2003) suggest that asthma is a form of airway obstruction that is reversible.

Bassett and Makin (2000) suggest that 2000 deaths occur each year in the UK as a result of asthma, 70% of which could be prevented by long-term therapy, assessment skills, and appropriate nursing care and management. Thirty per cent of the patients who die as a result of asthma do so within 2 hours of the onset of an attack.

Altered physiology

Bronchospasm occurs as a result of contraction of the smooth muscle. Inflammation happens and this causes hypersensitivity of the airways, which narrow as the result of a wide range of stimuli. Inflammatory cells cause even more narrowing of the airways.

Predisposing factors (triggers)

There are certain factors that can trigger an asthmatic attack. Cutler and Murch (2003) suggest that asthma trigger factors include:

- allergies, e.g. to pollen or house-dust mites
- infection, e.g. colds or other viral infections
- emotions, e.g. crying
- environment, e.g. tobacco smoke, pollution.

Signs and symptoms

- The patient may complain of a 'tight chest' or the feeling of suffocation.
- Breathing starts to increase in rate; there is exaggeration of the accessory muscle of respiration, with an audible wheeze on expiration.
- The patient may become distressed, wanting to sit upright.
- Accessory muscles are used to force air out.
- There is a tachycardia.
- The chest becomes hyperexpanded with some evidence of peripheral cyanosis.
- There will be a lower PEFR than the patient is 'normally' able to produce (if the patient can produce a PEFR).
- The inflammatory response may result in the production of thick mucoid sputum.
- The event can last for 1 hour to several days, resulting in central cyanosis, exhaustion, dehydration and eventually respiratory failure.

Diagnosis

Diagnosis is based on the patient's history of his or her present condition; the nurse must ensure that he or she does not exacerbate the patient's condition by asking questions that will make the patient's breathlessness worse. Data may need to be obtained from a significant other, another health-care professional or the patient's notes. The nurse's questioning technique will have to be sensitive to the patient's condition.

The nurse must have acute observational skills for observing the patient's posture, verbal and non-verbal signs. A chest radiograph may demonstrate pulmonary consolidation. Respiratory effort will be decreased and SaO_2 may fall below 95%. The nurse must record observations in the patient's notes and report any abnormalities.

Nursing interventions

The nurse must show that she or he is calm and in control, and act in a reassuring manner. The patient should be sat in the upright position or a position that he or she finds comfortable in order to increase thoracic capacity. Then the following interventions may be carried out:

- Administer all treatment as prescribed
- Remove, if possible, the allergen, e.g. if the patient is allergic to feathers ensure that the pillow is not made of feathers
- Oxygen therapy
- Salbutamol nebulizer
- Ipratropium bromide nebulizer
- Aminophylline (bronchodilator)
- Hydrocortisone (steroid with anti-inflammatory properties)
- Antibiotics
- Intravenous fluids.

Patient education

Specifically, the patient will need to be made aware of the possible triggers that may cause an asthmatic attack. The nurse needs to ensure that the patient is using the correct inhaler technique; if, despite repeated attempts to teach the patient the correct technique, the performance does not improve, the nurse should consider another inhaler delivery system, e.g. a volumatic or breath-actuated device (Johnson et al. 2000). The patient will need to be told what to do if he or she experiences another asthma attack. It is important that the patient has an adequate supply of inhalers at home and at work in case he or she needs to use them in order to relieve symptoms.

Chronic obstructive pulmonary disease

Chronic obstructive pulmonary disease (COPD) is an umbrella term applied to diseases such as chronic bronchitis, emphysema and asthma, which may result in permanent airway restriction. According to Bassett (2003), 99% of people who have COPD have smoked or are still smoking.

COPD is the world's fourth leading cause of disease-related death, killing 3 million people a year; it can mean a life of disability for the patient (Shamash 2000). As a result of the permanent reduction in airflow, patients will become reliant on lower levels of O_2 and higher levels of CO_2 to stimulate breathing. This is known as a hypoxic drive. It is vital that care is taken when delivering prescribed O_2.

Altered physiology

The disease spectrum varies widely from total obstructive airway disease with bronchitis to severe emphysema without bronchitis. The pathophysiological processes that cause the changes associated with pulmonary disease are neither static nor necessarily progressive (Phipps 1995). The altered physiology therefore depends on the underlying disease process.

To treat the patient appropriately and successfully, the nurse must determine what the underlying pulmonary disease is that is causing the patient's individual COPD. Often COPD is divided into key areas, e.g. chronic bronchitis, emphysema and asthma.

Caring for a patient with asthma was discussed earlier. The following subsections briefly outline the signs and symptoms, nursing interventions and related patient education associated with chronic bronchitis because the clinical manifestations for both chronic bronchitis and emphysema are similar.

Chronic bronchitis: signs and symptoms

Chronic bronchitis is often associated with the inhalation of physical or chemical irritants; cigarette smoking is by far the major risk factor in chronic bronchitis (Smeltzer and Bare 2000). The effect of the irritants on the airways results in hypersecretion of mucus and inflammation. Exacerbations of chronic bronchitis are most likely to occur during the winter months. The symptoms are:

- productive cough (especially on waking)
- chest infection (pyrexia, tachycardia)
- shortness of breath, dyspnoea
- cyanosis (central/peripheral).

Chronic bronchitis: diagnosis

To make a diagnosis of chronic bronchitis the nurse needs to obtain a full history of the present condition; he or she also needs to include a family history and to ascertain whether the patient has been exposed to any environmental factors such as tobacco, air pollution or occupational exposure to hazardous airborne materials. An in-depth holistic assessment is required gathering both subjective and objective data. The following investigations are also needed to make a definitive diagnosis:

- chest radiograph
- arterial blood gas analysis
- respiratory rate, rhythm and depth
- temperature
- pulse oximetry
- pulmonary function studies
- venous blood analysis
- sputum studies for microscopy, culture and sensitivity.

Chronic bronchitis: nursing interventions

The key aim of nursing care is to try to keep the bronchioles open and functioning in order to prevent infection and remove secretions. The nurse must assist the patient to carry out the activities of living so as not to exacerbate the condition. Regular measurement of vital signs is imperative; these must be recorded and abnormalities reported. A multidisciplinary approach is advocated and the nurse should act as the pivot for such an approach. Observation of any sputum must be made by the nurse and he or she should note and report any change in colour, amount and tenacity.

- Nurse the patient upright (unless contraindicated); encourage the patient to rest to conserve energy.
- Provide the patient with regular opportunities to clean the mouth because he or she may be mouth breathing; place tissues, sputum pot and a bag in which to put the used tissues within easy reach.
- Prevent cross-infection by restricting visits from people who have respiratory infections; encourage the patient to use tissues when dealing with his or her own secretions.
- Administer and report the effectiveness of any prescribed bronchodilators.
- Administer prescribed antibiotic therapy.
- Administer prescribed steroid therapy.
- Administer the prescribed amount of oxygen with humidification.
- Ensure that the patient is appropriately hydrated with oral fluids or intravenous fluids (correct hydration will help to loosen secretions and encourage expectoration).
- The nurse must ensure that he or she explains about treatment and nursing care to the patient in a way that he or she will understand.

Chronic bronchitis: patient education

Every effort should be made by the nurse working in conjunction with the patient, the family and if need be the employer to prevent recurrence of the condition (Smeltzer and Bare 2000). Those who are prone to respiratory tract infections should be given information that will enable them to make the decision about taking the vaccine against influenza and *Streptococcus pneumoniae* (Phipps 1995). The patient should be encouraged to give up smoking and avoid respiratory irritants and infections. In some instances, the patient will need to undergo an occupational health assessment at his or her place of work.

The nurse may need to teach/reinforce the correct method of using nebulizers or inhalers at home. It is important that the patient understands the reasons for the prescribed medications. Instil in the patient the signs that may necessitate seeking nursing/medical attention should another episode of illness occur, because often antimicrobial therapy should be started at the first sign of purulent sputum.

Conclusions

This chapter has provided the nurse with the underlying physiological, anatomical and nursing concepts to help the provision of high-quality care that is commensurate with the requirements laid down by the Nursing and Midwifery Council (NMC 2000). It has also provided the nurse with the fundamental concepts and the reader is urged to delve further in order to improve on knowledge and thus nursing care.

Caring for a patient with a respiratory disorder requires skilled nursing care in order to assess, plan, implement and evaluate appropriate nursing interventions. The nurse must be an effective communicator in order to communicate with patients and family, who are often distressed, anxious and fearful. The nurse needs to have a good understanding of the anatomy and physiology of the respiratory tract, in order to make clinical decisions that are based on fact as opposed to hearsay or tradition.

The assessment of respiratory function is complex. The maintenance of optimum oxygenation in patients with respiratory tract disorders is a key priority for nurses in both hospital and community settings.

This chapter has briefly introduced the nurse to many key nursing skills, and the skills required to assess the patient's respiratory needs have been discussed in some detail. By understanding and using the information provided the nurse will be able to perform in a more effective manner, respond appropriately and enhance the quality of care that he or she provides.

The nurse needs to be able to detect any abnormalities quickly and to act on his or her findings. It is advocated that the nurse should record and report any changes in the patient's condition. Ongoing assessment and evaluation of nursing interventions are vital in order to respond quickly to changing situations, which may have implications for patient outcomes.

References

Asthma Training Centre (1997) The Asthma Training Centre Learning Package. Stratford upon Avon: Asthma Training Centre.

Baillie, L., Corben, V. and Higham, C. (2001) Respiratory care: Assessment and interventions. In: Baillie, L. (ed.), Developing Practical Nursing Skills. London: Arnold, pp. 285–332.

Bassett, C. (ed.) (2003) Essentials of Nursing Care. London: Whurr Publishers.

Bassett, C. and Makin, L. (2000) Caring for the Seriously Ill Patient. London: Arnold.

Brewin, A. (1997) Comparing asthma and chronic obstructive pulmonary disease (COPD). Nursing Standard 12(4): 49–55.

Cutler, L. and Murch, P. (2003) The respiratory system. In: Bassett, C. (ed.), Essentials of Nursing Care. London: Whurr Publishers, pp. 47–92.

Daniels, R. (2002) Delmar's Guide to Laboratory and Diagnostic Tests. New York: Delmar.

Epstein, O., Perkin, G.D., de Bono, D.P. and Cookson, J. (1997) Clinical Examination, 2nd edn. London: Mosby.

Grandis, S., Long, C., Glasper, A. and Jackson, P. (2003) Foundation Studies for Nursing: Using enquiry-based learning. Basingstoke: Palgrave Macmillan.

Hogston, R. and Simpson, P.M. (2002) Foundations of Nursing Practice: Making a difference, 2nd edn. Basingstoke: Palgrave Macmillan.

Jenkins, J. (2003) Breathing. In: Holland, K., Jenkins, J., Solomon, J. and Whittam, S. (eds), Applying the Roper, Logan and Tierney Model in Practice. Edinburgh: Churchill Livingstone, pp. 121–161.

Johnson, G., Hill-Smith, I. and Ellis, C. (2000) The Minor Illness Manual, 2nd edn. Oxford: Radcliffe Medical Press.

Law, C. (2000) A guide to assessing sputum. Nursing Times 96(24): 7–10.

McEwing, G., Kelsey, J., Richardson, J. and Glasper, A. (2003) Insights into child and family health. In: Grandis, S., Long, C., Glasper, A. and Jackson, P. (eds), Foundation Studies for Nursing: Using enquiry-based learning. Basingstoke: Palgrave, pp. 48–114.

Mallett, J. and Dougherty, L. (2000) Royal Marsden Hospital Manual of Clinical Nursing Procedures, 5th edn. Oxford: Blackwell Science.

Marieb, E.N. (2004) Human Anatomy and Physiology, 6th edn. London: Pearson Benjamin Cummings.

Martini, F.H. (2001) Fundamentals of Anatomy and Physiology, 5th edn. London: Mosby.

Nicol, M., Bavin, C., Bedford-Turner, S., Cronin, P. and Rawlings-Anderson, K. (2000) Essential Nursing Skills. Edinburgh: Mosby.

Nursing and Midwifery Council (2000) Code of Professional Conduct. London: NMC.

Phipps, W.J. (1995) The patient with pulmonary problems. In: Long, B.C., Phipps, W.J. and Cassmeyer, V.L. (eds), Adult Nursing: A nursing process approach. London: Mosby, pp. 510–630.

Roper, N., Logan, W.W. and Tierney, A.J. (1996) The Elements of Nursing: A model for nursing based on a model for living, 4th edn. Edinburgh: Churchill Livingstone.

Roper, N., Logan, W.W. and Tierney, A.J. (2000) The Roper, Logan and Tierney Model of Nursing Based on Activities of Living. Edinburgh: Churchill Livingstone.

Sadik, R. and Elliott, D. (2002) Respiration and circulation. In: Hogston, R. and Simpson, P.M. (eds), Foundations of Nursing Practice: Making the difference. London: Palgrave, pp. 185–237.

Shamash, J. (2000) Catching their breath. Nursing Times 98(20): 14.

Smeltzer, S.C. and Bare, B.G. (2000) Brunner and Suddarth's Textbook of Medical–Surgical Nursing. Philadelphia: Lippincott.

Street, M. (2003) The cardiovascular system. In: Bassett, C. (ed.), Essentials of Nursing Care. London: Whurr Publishers, pp. 1–46.

Walsh, M. (2002) Watson's Clinical Nursing and Related Sciences, 6th edn. London: Baillière Tindall.

Whittaker, N. (2004) Chronic obstructive pulmonary disease (COPD). In: Whittaker, N. (ed.), Disorders and Interventions. London: Palgrave, pp. 201–232.

Woolons, S. (1995) Peak flow meters. Professional Nurse 11: 130–132.

CHAPTER 6

Eating and drinking: nutrient and fluid requirements for health

JANE SAY

This chapter considers the body's requirements for nutrients and fluids to maintain good health. It is hoped that by understanding these principles you will be able to deliver the care required for those patients who have particular care needs to maintain their eating and drinking requirements.

Good nutrition is essential to the maintenance of health throughout our lives. It has long been recognized that poor nutrition can lead to ill-health. A wealth of research exists that links different aspects of our dietary intakes with illness and disease processes (Department of Health [DoH] 1991, 1998, Puska et al. 1995).

Also vital to our health is the body's fluid balance. Principally our body fluids comprise water and a number of solutes (chemicals that can dissolve in water). Within the body the composition and distribution of our body fluids are carefully maintained so that the environment around our cells is consistent. To maintain water balance, water intake must equal water output (Marieb 2004). Without adequate fluid intake dehydration will occur and ultimately cellular activity will be disrupted. Death will occur in extreme dehydration.

Within clinical practice several different members of the multidisciplinary team (MDT) will be involved in ensuring the nutrient and fluid intakes of adult clients. These may include:

- doctors
- dietitians
- nutritional nurse specialists
- pharmacists
- occupational therapists
- speech and language therapists.

Within this context nurses have a pivotal role in promoting and maintaining nutritional and fluid intakes. To fulfil this important function

92

nurses must have an understanding of both the components of a healthy diet and the fluid requirements of their clients. They must also be able to assess and monitor the nutritional and fluid status of their clients, and they should be able to deliver and monitor special therapeutic diets and fluid replacement. Nurses also have a duty of care and must act in the patient's best interests at all times (Nursing and Midwifery Council [NMC] 2002). Finally, nurses must be able to work effectively within the MDT to ensure that the most appropriate care is given to their clients.

What is nutrition?

Nutrition is a combination of processes by which cells receive and use food material or nutrients to support and maintain metabolism in all parts of the body.

Nutrients in food can be split into two broad categories: macro-nutrients and micronutrients. The macronutrients are those that provide energy and include carbohydrates, fats, proteins and alcohol. Fibre (also known as non-starch polysaccharide or NSP) is also classed as a macronutrient, although pure fibre does not provide energy for the body. Micronutrients constitute vitamins, minerals and trace elements. They have a wide range of functions but, unlike the macronutrients, do not provide energy for the body.

Both macro- and micronutrients are used by chemical reactions that occur in the body. These reactions form the body's metabolism and occur at a cellular level. A specific amount of both major types of nutrients is required if normal cellular functioning is to occur.

Nutritional requirements

Within the UK, the requirements for both macro- and micronutrients have been determined by the Committee on Medical Aspects of Food Policy (COMA) (DoH 1991). This group used scientific evidence to determine the nutritional requirements of different people within the population. These guidelines for nutrient intakes replaced the old recommended dietary allowances (RDA). For each key nutrient within the diet the Committee determined a range of intakes that would ensure that the requirements of the whole population and individuals within the population were being met. The term used for this range is the 'dietary reference value' (DRV). Within clinical practice, dietitians and those within the catering department use these figures to ensure that the diet of individual clients, and the client population as a whole, are being considered. For further details on the definitions determined by the COMA report and their key recommendations, refer to the Health Education Authority's *Synopsis of Dietary Reference Values* (HEA 1996).

The macronutrients

Energy requirements

Carbohydrates, fats, proteins and alcohol all provide the body with the raw nutrients required to generate energy. Fats contain the most calories (9 kilocalories per gram or kcal/g), whereas carbohydrates contain 3.75 kcal/g and proteins 4 kcal/g.

The body needs energy to maintain our normal metabolic activity even at rest. This ensures that the body can function normally. However, energy is also needed to meet our extra needs for physical activity and work. If our energy intake matches our energy needs, we will maintain a constant weight. As you might expect, energy requirements alter throughout life and are related to age, sex, race and levels of physical activity. Hence, a young male soldier who is busy training will have much higher requirements for energy than an older woman who is immobile. Children, for their height and weight, have high demands for energy as a result of their requirements for normal growth and development. Table 6.1 gives the average energy requirements for different groups of people in the population.

Table 6.1 Estimated average energy requirements of different population groups (DoH 1991)

Age	Males MJ/day (kcal/day)	Females MJ/day (kcal/day)
0–3 months	2.28 (545)	2.16 (515)
4–6 months	2.89 (690)	2.69 (645)
7–9 months	3.44 (825)	3.20 (765)
10–12 months	3.85 (690)	3.61 (865)
1–3 years	5.2 (1230)	4.9 (1165)
4–6 years	7.2 (1715)	6.5 (1545)
7–10 years	8.2 (1970)	7.3 (1740)
11–14 years	9.3 (2220)	7.9 (1845)
15–18 years	11.5 (2755)	8.8 (2110)
Adults	10.6 (2550)	8.0 (1940)
75+ years	8.77 (2100)	7.61 (1810)

Carbohydrates

This term describes a group of compounds that contain the chemicals carbon, hydrogen and oxygen. Starch and sugars are carbohydrates that can be used to provide energy for the body. NSP (dietary fibre) does not provide energy but can perform a number of other functions within the body.

Sugars

These are soluble carbohydrates and can be monosaccharides (single sugar units, e.g. glucose, fructose and ribose) or disaccharides (double sugar units, e.g. sucrose, lactose and maltose). They can be further described as intrinsic sugars or extrinsic sugars:

- *Intrinsic sugars* are found within the cellular structure of some unprocessed foods such as fruit and vegetables.
- *Extrinsic sugars* are not found within the cellular structure of foods. There are two types of these sugars:
  - milk sugars occurring naturally in milk and milk products
  - non-milk extrinsic sugars, which include recipe and table sugars.

It is recommended that the amount of non-milk extrinsic sugars in our diets be reduced. These sugars, which are found in cakes, soft drinks and sweets, and are added to recipes, cause tooth decay and can cause people to become overweight or obese (HEA 1996).

Starch

This is found in bread, cereals and root vegetables; such foods are often rich in NSPs. Starch is a polysaccharide and as such is made up of long chains of sugar units. Within our diet it is an important means of providing energy and the COMA (DoH 1991) report recommends an increase in consumption of fibre-rich starchy foods.

Glycogen

This is an important polysaccharide within humans and is made up of long chains of glucose molecules. It forms the main storage carbohydrate in the body and is found in the liver and muscles.

Non-starch polysaccharide (dietary fibre)

Non-starch polysaccharide, or fibre as it is more commonly known, is an essential part of a healthy diet. There are two types of NSP, each with slightly different properties. Water-soluble NSPs found in oats, pulses and fruit may lower blood cholesterol, and reduce postprandial (after a meal) blood glucose and triglyceride levels. Water-insoluble NSPs aid the amount of faeces produced, which reduces the incidence of constipation and can lead to a reduction in diseases such as diverticulitis and bowel cancer (Kromhout et al. 1982).

Fats

Fats or lipids include a wide range of dietary components and fatty substances. Like the carbohydrates, they principally contain carbon, hydrogen and oxygen, but in different proportions to carbohydrates. The major dietary fats are triglycerides, cholesterol and fatty acids. Triglycerides are composed of a glycerol molecule attached to three fatty acids. There are three main types of fatty acid: saturated fatty acids (SFAs), monounsaturated fatty acids (MUFAs) and polyunsaturated fatty acids (PUFAs). All foods contain a mixture of fatty acids.

Saturated fatty acids

These contain a chain of carbon atoms that is saturated with hydrogen atoms. They are found mainly in foods of animal origin and dairy products such as hard margarine and butter. Products made from these, such as cakes, pastries, pies and biscuits, will have saturated fats within them. Increased intakes of these fatty acids can cause an increase in the body's serum (within the bloodstream) cholesterol levels. Increased cholesterol levels can lead to coronary heart disease and atherosclerosis (fat deposition in the arteries leading to narrowing and occlusion of blood flow) (DoH 1994).

Monounsaturated fatty acids

These have a carbon chain that has one double bond between carbon atoms. This means that it is not completely saturated by hydrogen atoms. Olive oil and rapeseed oil contain a lot of monounsaturates, but they are also found in meat and dairy produce. These fatty acids are believed to protect against the development of coronary heart disease and are found in large amounts in Mediterranean diets where the incidence of heart disease is low (DoH 1994).

Polyunsaturated fatty acids

These molecules have a carbon chain, but it is not saturated by hydrogen atoms. They contain a number of 'double bonds'. Polyunsaturates are principally found in vegetable oils such as maize, soya bean and sunflower oil. Two PUFAs (linoleic acid and linolenic acid) are classed as essential fatty acids because they cannot be synthesized in the body and must therefore be provided in the diet.

Overall, there are two main types of PUFA, which are called omega-3 (ω-3 or *n*-3) and omega-6 (ω-6 or *n*-6) fatty acids. Omega-3 fatty acids have been found to reduce the risk of a second myocardial infarction (MI or heart attack). This is because they reduce the tendency for the blood to clot. They are believed to be beneficial against cardiovascular disease (CVD) and they are needed for fetal development (DoH 1994, Scientific Advisory Committee on Nutrition [SACN] 2004). As such it is recommended that two portions of fish should be eaten each week, one of which should be an oily fish. Despite recent concerns about toxins within fish, and particularly oily fish, these recommendations have recently been endorsed by the SACN (2004). Pregnant women are advised not to eat shark, swordfish or marlin because they may contain high levels of toxins that are harmful to their fetus.

Cholesterol

This is found in foods of mainly animal origin. Cholesterol can be synthesized by the liver from saturated fatty acids.

Although the main function of lipids within the body is to provide energy, it should be noted that fats have a number of other important roles in the body. Triglycerides are stored as a reserve of energy within adipose tissue and these stores act as a means of insulation, protection and cushioning for the body. Cholesterol is needed to make bile salts and steroid hormones (e.g. oestrogen and testosterone) and forms an important structural component within the plasma membrane that surrounds all cells. PUFAs are also important for the plasma membrane and are needed to synthesize chemicals called prostaglandins (which are important for the immune system and other aspects of body function).

Proteins

Proteins are very important in the diet because they are essential for the proper structure and function of the body. Proteins are found in meat, fish, eggs and dairy produce. They are also found in pulses (peas, beans and lentils), nuts, tofu and soya, and in cereal products such as bread and pasta. The building blocks of proteins are amino acids. Within the body 20 amino acids combine in many different ways to form the thousands of different proteins found in the body. These amino acids are composed from carbon, hydrogen and oxygen, and in addition the elements nitrogen, sulphur and phosphate.

The proteins that form the body can be categorized into two main groups: structural proteins and functional proteins.

Structural proteins

These include actin and myosin (which are found in muscle tissue) and collagen (important for the structure of the skin and other organs in the body).

Functional proteins

These include enzymes that control chemical reactions, antibodies that protect against disease, hormones that control cellular processes and the blood proteins, such as albumin and haemoglobin (which is actually situated within red blood cells).

Some amino acids can be synthesized by the body as long as overall protein intake is sufficient. Those amino acids that are not needed in the diet are called 'non-essential amino acids'. However, there are several amino acids that cannot be synthesized. These are termed 'essential amino acids' and must be included in the diet.

Protein requirements vary according to age and gender. Certain foods have a high biological value for proteins and contain all the essential amino acids. Such foods are normally from animal food sources. Foods from most vegetable sources (except soya) tend to be of a lower biological value.

Alcohol

Alcohol is also made up of carbon, hydrogen and oxygen. It has a high calorific value of 7 kcal/g. This high calorific value means that increased intakes on a regular basis can lead to obesity. Excessive intakes of alcohol can also lead to serious illness and death. Long-term abuse can cause both physical and psychological addiction.

However, alcohol in moderation can have a protective effect against coronary heart disease (DoH 1995). Alcohol intake is measured in units, with each unit containing 8 g pure alcohol. The Department of Health (1995) recommends that women can drink only up to 2–3 units per day (except during pregnancy) and men only up to 3–4 units per day; binge drinking should be avoided.

The micronutrients

The micronutrients are essential for human nutrition but are required in very small amounts. They have a number of functions in the body and can be classified as vitamins and minerals. Vitamins are organic compounds (i.e. they contain carbon) whereas minerals are inorganic elements that are also needed by the body (Bender 2002).

The activity of the micronutrients within the body varies greatly. Many are important in cellular metabolism and function. Some micronutrients act as co-factors to enzymes whereas others act as activators of enzymes. Many of the dietary vitamins have roles as co-factors to enzyme activity. Both co-factors and activators enable enzyme activity to occur. Enzymes are biological catalysts that speed up the rate of chemical reactions, and without their activity the chemical reactions of the body would not proceed quickly enough for normal body function. As a consequence, deficiencies of those micronutrients that influence enzyme activity will lead to the disruption of normal cellular metabolism.

Other micronutrients have important structural and functional roles within tissues and certain specialized proteins in the body. Calcium (a mineral) forms a key structural component of bone because it is deposited as calcium salts within the matrix of the bone tissue. Iron (another mineral) is an essential component of the red blood cell protein haemoglobin. Iron is required for haemoglobin to bind with oxygen and thus maintains the function of the red blood cells.

Another group of micronutrients is termed 'antioxidants' or 'free radical scavengers'. Free radicals are chemicals that are generated during normal metabolism. An example of how free radicals are formed in the body is during the process of phagocytosis in those white blood cells known as neutrophils. These cells engulf (or phagocytose) bacteria as a means of fighting infection. During this process, the neutrophils generate free radicals that then destroy the phagocytosed bacteria. However, free radicals can also cause unwanted damage to cells, and in particular they may damage the cell membranes that surround and protect cells. This will ultimately cause cell death. Free radicals may also affect the structure of deoxyribonucleic acid (DNA – the genetic material within cells). Such changes in DNA can ultimately give rise to the development of malignant tumours. Free radical scavengers or antioxidants have the ability to protect cells and tissues from this sort of damage.

Sodium, potassium and chloride are important minerals within the body. The special properties of these minerals within solution mean that they are also called electrolytes. They have essential roles in body fluid and acid–base balance, and are also essential for nerve and muscle conduction.

For details of the estimated average reference (EAR) values of the different micronutrients, refer to the COMA report (DoH 1991). Table 6.2 outlines the key functions and sources of the micronutrients.

A diet for health

A healthy eating pattern requires the correct balance of macro- and micronutrients. A healthy diet is composed of a range and combination of foods. A means of obtaining the right amount of nutrients is to select the foods as suggested in Table 6.3. This food selection is based on the five key food groups that make a significant contribution to our diet. This guide is based on the recommendations within *The Balance of Good Health*. It was developed by the Health Education Authority, the Department of Health and the Ministry of Agriculture, Fisheries and Food (HEA et al. 1994). It is designed to promote healthy eating in a simple and understandable way.

This guide is intended for the majority of the population. This includes those with a desired weight for height (normal body mass index or BMI – a discussion of this is included Chapter 7), vegetarians and people of all ethnic origins. Children under the age of 2 years (because they need full fat milk and dairy products), elderly people and those who are ill may have different requirements. Children between 2 and 5 years should make a gradual transition to this style of diet. It is recommended that people under medical supervision always seek further medical advice about following this guide.

This guide also supports the government's guidelines for healthy eating. These are:

1. Enjoy your food
2. Eat a varied diet to meet vitamin and mineral requirements
3. Eat the right amount to be a healthy weight

Table 6.2 Micronutrients in the body

Vitamin	Source	Function	Deficiency	Excess
A	Dairy foods, fish liver oils, liver, carrots and leafy green vegetables	Essential for retinal pigments in the eye that maintain normal vision; growth and integrity of epithelial tissues, bones and teeth	Delayed growth; blindness; changes to epithelial tissues including the skin; infections	High intakes have been associated with birth defects and as such pregnant women are advised not to take supplements of vitamin A
D	Egg yolk, fish liver oils (can be added to milk and margarine). Also naturally produced in the skin on exposure to UV rays (sunlight)	Increases calcium levels by aiding calcium absorption. Ensures normal development of bones and teeth and is important for blood clotting and neuromuscular activity	Rickets in children and osteomalacia in adults. Poor muscle tone, restlessness and irritability	High doses can cause toxicity. Symptoms include vomiting, hypercalcaemia and calcification of soft tissues
E	Wheat germ, vegetable oils, nuts, whole grains and leafy green vegetables	Antioxidant that protects cell membranes from damage by free radicals	Effects are uncertain. Pre-term infants are at risk as a result of low reserves of vitamin E. Haemolytic anaemia may occur as a result of the membranes of red blood cells being attacked by free radicals	Few side effects at high doses
K	Synthesized in the large intestine by bacteria. Also found in leafy vegetables, broccoli, cabbage and cauliflower	Essential for the synthesis of a number of blood clotting proteins	Easy bruising and bleeding/prolonged clotting time	None known
Thiamine (B$_1$)	Meat, liver, fish, eggs and leafy vegetables	Acts as a coenzyme and is important for carbohydrate metabolism in the body	Disease called beri-beri caused by long-term deficiency. Wernicke–Korsakoff syndrome associated with acute deficiency and often seen in alcoholics. Muscle weakness, atrophy and heart failure are associated with deficiency.	None known

Cont.

	Sources	Function	Deficiency	Toxicity/excess
			Wernicke–Korsakoff syndrome is characterized by short-term memory loss and central nervous system damage	
Riboflavin (B$_2$)	Wide sources, including: liver, yeast, egg whites, meat, grains, poultry and dairy produce	Acts as a coenzyme and is important for the metabolism of carbohydrates, fats and proteins	Dermatitis, cracking at the edge of lips (cheilosis) and corners of the mouth (angular stomatitis). Skin lesions and changes in the epithelia of the tongue also occur	None known
Niacin	Proteins are a good source of niacin	Acts as a coenzyme and is important for the metabolism of carbohydrates, fats and proteins	The disease pellagra is caused by deficiency. This can lead to dermatitis, diarrhoea, dementia and death	High levels can cause flushing, potential liver damage and skin irritation
Pyridoxine (B$_6$)	Meat, poultry, fish and bananas	Acts as a coenzyme and is important for the metabolism of carbohydrates, fats and proteins	Clinical deficiency is rare. In infants, convulsions may occur	High intakes over a long period can cause damage to peripheral nerves
Folate/folic acid	Liver, yeast extracts and green leafy vegetables.	Needed for coenzymes associated with amino acid metabolism and DNA synthesis. Important for neural tube development in early pregnancy	Deficiency affects cells that are rapidly dividing. Signs of deficiency may include megaloblastic anaemia (resulting from effects on red blood cell production) and diarrhoea (caused by the effects on the intestinal mucosa). Inadequate folic acid nutrition in expectant mothers can cause spina bifida and congenital neural tube defects. Supplements before conception and during the first 3 months of pregnancy can significantly reduce this happening	None known

Table 6.2 *Cont.*

Vitamin	Source	Function	Deficiency	Excess
B_{12}	Liver, meat, poultry, some dairy foods and fish	Important as a coenzyme in the synthesis of DNA. Important for normal function of the gastrointestinal tract, bone marrow and the nervous system	Deficiency is usually a result of lack of absorption from the gastrointestinal tract. To be absorbed, a protein (called intrinsic factor) produced by the cells of the stomach is needed. Failure to secrete intrinsic factor causes vitamin B_{12} deficiency. Deficiency causes megaloblastic anaemia and rarely can cause degeneration of the spinal cord	None known
Biotin	Widely distributed in foods including liver, egg yolk and nuts	Needed for coenzymes associated with carbohydrate, fat and protein metabolism	Extremely rare. Symptoms include: scaly skin, muscle pains, anorexia and nausea	None known
Pantothenic acid	Widely distributed in all foods	Needed for coenzyme A. This facilitates carbohydrate, fat and protein metabolism	Extremely rare. Symptoms include fatigue, headache, dizziness, muscle weakness and gastrointestinal tract disturbances	None known
C	Fruits and vegetables, particularly citrus fruits	Antioxidant that protects cell membranes from damage by free radicals. Important for the formation of connective tissues (including collagen) and as such has an important role in wound healing. Also enhances iron absorption from the gastrointestinal tract	Scurvy is the disease associated with vitamin C deficiency. The effects on collagen synthesis cause problems with the gums and teeth and can delay wound healing. Disruption to hair follicles also occurs. Susceptibility to infection and bone pain are further consequences of deficiency	Possible effects of high intakes include diarrhoea and kidney stones

Mineral	Source	Function	Deficiency	Excess
Calcium	Milk, milk products, leafy green vegetables, egg yolk, shellfish	Essential for healthy bones and teeth. Needed for nerve and muscle activity	Tetany, osteomalacia, osteoporosis. Retarded growth and rickets in children	Lethargy and confusion, kidney stones, depressed neural function
Iron	Meat, liver and shellfish	Forms part of the haem group in haemoglobin. This binds oxygen in the red blood cells	Iron deficiency anaemia. Causes pallor, lethargy, anorexia and impaired cognitive ability in children	Haemochromatosis (inherited condition where there is excessive iron in the body). Can cause damage to liver, heart and pancreas
Potassium	Widely distributed in foods	Needed for normal nerve and muscle activity. Helps to maintain the normal composition of blood, intracellular fluid and extracellular fluid	Hypokalaemia is rare, but may be seen in excessive diarrhoea and vomiting or as a side effect of certain drug therapies. Can cause cardiac arrhythmias and cardiac arrest. Also muscle paralysis or weakness	Hyperkalaemia is usually a complication of renal failure or particular drug therapies. Cardiac arrhythmias can result from this
Sodium	Found in table salts and added in foods	Needed for normal nerve and muscle activity. Helps to maintain the water balance along with the normal composition of blood, intracellular fluid and extracellular fluid	Hyponatraemia is rare, but may be seen in excessive diarrhoea, vomiting and sweating or if a client is over-hydrated	Hypernatraemia may be seen in dehydrated clients. Excessive salt intakes can lead to hypertension
Zinc	Seafoods, meat, cereals, yeast and wheat germ	Important for the function of several enzymes. Required for normal growth, wound healing, taste, smell and sperm production	Loss of taste, immune suppression, delayed wound healing, delayed puberty and decreased sperm production	Difficulty in walking, slurred speech and tremors
Chlorine	Found in table salts and added in foods	Exists as chloride ion in the body. Found mainly in extracellular fluid. Helps to maintain the water balance along with the normal pH of blood	Severe vomiting or diarrhoea leads to chloride loss and can lead to changes in acid-base balance	Vomiting

Table 6.3 The five key nutrients and recommendations for health

Food group	Bread, cereals and potatoes	Fruit and vegetables	Milk and dairy foods	Meat, fish and alternatives	Foods containing fat and foods containing sugar
Food within the group	Cereals include things such as breakfast cereals, pasta, rice, oats, noodles, maize, millet and cornmeal	Fresh frozen and canned fruit and vegetables and dried fruit. A glass of fruit juice can also contribute. Beans and pulses can be eaten as part of this group	Milk, cheese, yoghurt and fromage frais. This group does not include butter, eggs and cream	Meat, poultry, fish, eggs, nuts, beans and pulses. Meat includes bacon and salami and meat products such as sausages, beef burgers and pâtés. These are all relatively high fat choices. Beans, such as canned baked beans and pulses, are in this group. Fish includes frozen and canned fish such as sardines and tuna, fish fingers and fish cakes	Foods containing fat: margarine, butter, other spreading fats and low-fat spreads, cooking oils, oil-based salad dressings, mayonnaise, cream, chocolate, crisps, biscuits, pastries, cake, puddings, ice-cream, rich sauces and gravies. Foods containing sugar: soft drinks, sweets, jam and sugar as well as foods such as cakes, puddings, biscuits, pastries and ice-cream
Key nutrients in the group	Carbohydrate (starch) Fibre (NSP) Some calcium and iron B vitamins	Vitamin C Carotenes Folates Fibre (NSP) and some carbohydrate	Calcium, zinc Protein Vitamins B_{12} and B_2 Vitamins A and D	Iron Protein B vitamins, especially vitamin B_{12} Zinc Magnesium	Fat, including some essential fatty acids, but also some vitamins. Some products also contain salt or sugar

| Recommendations | Eat lots | Eat lots | Eat or drink moderate amounts and choose lower-fat versions whenever you can | 'Lower-fat versions' means foods like meat with the fat cut off, poultry without the skin and fish without batter. Cook these foods without added fat. Beans and pulses are good alternatives to meat as they are naturally very low in fat | Eat foods containing fat sparingly and look out for the low-fat alternatives. Foods containing sugar should not be eaten too often as they can contribute to tooth decay |

Adapted from the Food Standards Agency (2001).

4. Eat plenty of foods rich in starch and fibre
5. Eat plenty of fruit and vegetables
6. Don't eat too many foods that contain a lot of fat
7. Don't have sugary foods and drinks too often
8. If you drink alcohol, drink sensibly.

Recently, in order to further this approach, more specific guidelines have been proposed by the government (DoH 2004). These are briefly outlined here:

• Energy intake from foods needs to balance with the energy used by the body. This helps to avoid obesity.
• The amount of fat in the overall diet of the population needs to be reduced because fats contain the most calories. Specifically the intake of saturated fat needs to be reduced.
• Alcohol also has a high calorie content and it can increase calorie intake. The public therefore needs to be aware of how much energy is contained in alcohol.
• To reduce calorific intakes and protect against tooth decay, the average intake of sugar (extrinsic sugars) needs to be reduced.
• The intake of dietary fibre needs to be increased.
• The average consumption of fruit and vegetables needs to be at least five portions per day.

To access further information on healthy eating please see the following websites:

• Food Standards Agency: www.foodstandards.gov.uk/aboutus/publications/
• British Nutrition Foundation: www.nutrition.org.uk/information/ dietandhealth/balanceddiet.html
• Weight Wise (developed by the British Dietetic Association): www. bdaweightwise.com

Body fluids and fluid balance

In the body, water accounts for about half the body mass. The amount of water in the body varies through the lifespan. In childhood water may account for as much as 73% of body mass whereas in old age this may only be 45%. In adulthood a healthy young man may have 60% body mass as water, whereas a healthy young female may have 50% (McCance and Huether 2002, Marieb 2004).

In the body, water is found in the following two main areas.

The intracellular fluid compartment

The intracellular fluid (ICF) is made up of all the cells in the body and this is where two-thirds of body water is found.

The extracellular fluid compartment

The remaining one-third of the body water is outside the cells, i.e. in the extracellular fluid (ECF). This is further divided into (1) the plasma (the fluid part of the bloodstream) and (2) the interstitial fluid (this is the fluid that surrounds the cells). Other fluid in the body, such as lymph, cerebrospinal fluid and secretions of the gastrointestinal tract, are included with the interstitial fluid. Table 6.4 shows the different fluid compartments in the body; these have been based on a 25-year-old 70-kg man.

Table 6.4 Distribution of fluid volumes in a 70-kg man

Total body water volume (42 litres (l) or 60% of body weight)			
Intracellular fluid volume 28 l or 40% of body weight	Extracellular fluid volume 14 l or 20% of body weight		
	Interstitial fluid volume 11.2 l or 80% of ECF	Plasma volume 2.8 l or 20% of ECF	

Composition of body fluids

Each of the body fluid compartments contains more than just water. Dissolved within the water are *electrolytes* and *non-electrolytes*. The nutrients that we eat are digested and absorbed into the plasma. These make up many of the electrolytes and non-electrolytes found in the plasma, e.g. potassium is a nutrient which, when dissolved in the plasma, forms an important electrolyte, whereas glucose when absorbed from the diet forms a key non-electrolyte in the plasma. Also found in the plasma are waste products of body metabolism, e.g. creatinine and urea. These are often non-electrolytes.

Electrolytes are chemicals that split into their component ions when they are dissolved in water, e.g. sodium chloride (in chemistry this salt, the same as table salt, is given the symbol NaCl) splits into a sodium ion (Na^+) and a chloride ion (Cl^-) when dissolved in water. These two ions have a charge: one is positively charged and one is negatively charged:

$$NaCl \rightarrow Na^+ + Cl^-$$

These charges, which form when electrolytes dissolve in water, allow the solution to conduct electricity. As such, body fluids have special properties and this is why nerve and muscle conduction can occur.

Non-electrolytes do not 'split' into ions when dissolved in water and therefore they do not conduct electricity.

Fluid movement and exchange in the body

Within the body there is a continuous exchange of water, electrolytes and non-electrolytes between the different fluid compartments.

Our blood plasma circulates throughout the body. Water, electrolytes and non-electrolytes (from the digestion of nutrients) enter the plasma from the gastrointestinal tract. Oxygen enters the plasma from the lungs. The blood plasma supplies the interstitial fluid and the ICF with the water and nutrients (including O_2) that the cells require to maintain metabolism. The cells generate a lot of waste products during metabolism. CO_2 leaves the cells and enters the plasma and from there it is removed from the body by the lungs. Other waste products such as creatinine and urea also leave the cells and enter the plasma. These are removed from the body by the kidneys.

Each fluid compartment of the body is not identical. The amount and type of electrolytes and non-electrolytes in the different compartments vary. However, the body controls the concentration of the body fluids very carefully by controlling the electrolytes and non-electrolytes in the body, and of course the amount of water in the body.

Water and fluid balance in the body

To maintain *fluid balance* the amount of water entering the body must be the same as the amount leaving it. Of course in normal health, drinking and eating are the methods by which we take in water. A small amount is also made by metabolic activity in the cells. However, there are several different ways that the body loses water. The most obvious loss is from the kidneys in the urine and from the gastrointestinal tract in the faeces. However, a significant amount of water is lost from the skin (through perspiration) and from the respiratory tract as we exhale.

Table 6.5 shows the average intake and output of water in an adult. Note that these values can vary between individuals. These may also change on a daily basis. Exercise and an increase in temperature on a hot day can drastically increase the amount of water lost via the skin through perspiration.

Table 6.5 The average water intake and output in adults

Intake	Volume (ml/day)	Output	Volume (ml/day)
Drinking	1200	Insensible loss	
		Skin	500
		Respiration	400
Eating	1000	Urine	1400
Metabolic activity	200	Faeces	100
Total	2400	Total	2400

The body has a number of methods to help to maintain our intake and output in order to ensure that the body fluids remain at the right concentration.

Water intake

When the body fluids become too concentrated because the body requires more water, the mouth becomes dry and the *thirst mechanism* occurs. The amount of saliva is reduced and higher centres in the brain (in an area called the hypothalamus) also trigger a feeling of thirst. Drinking water helps to satisfy the thirst.

Water output

It has been demonstrated that each day we will lose a certain amount of water from the body regardless of our intake. This water loss is called obligatory (which means it must occur). Part of this loss is the insensible loss from our skin and lungs and the water loss in our faeces. In addition, each day our kidneys must excrete approximately 500 ml of water to ensure that the waste products that are constantly produced in the body are expelled.

The water excreted from the kidney over and above the obligatory 500 ml is variable and depends on our fluid intake and diet on the day. It is also affected by how much fluid is lost in other ways, e.g. increased perspiration on a hot day will increase water loss. As such the kidneys would reduce the amount of water they excrete. Similarly, during a period of diarrhoea the body will lose significantly more water via the faeces and as such the kidneys will excrete less water. Within the body there are a number of hormonal mechanisms that affect water and electrolyte balance.

Conclusion

Within this chapter aspects of nutrition and the nutritional requirements of our bodies have been explored. These included the nature of the macro- and micronutrients and their functions within the body. Consideration was also given to the components of a healthy diet in the light of current government recommendations.

The body's requirements for water and the need for fluid balance have also been considered. This knowledge helps to inform and underpin nursing practice when dealing with issues related to eating and drinking.

In Chapter 7 these principles are applied and developed in relation to managing patients' fluid and nutritional needs, and maintaining their health through the processes of eating and drinking.

References

Bender, D.A. (2002) Introduction to Nutrition and Metabolism, 3rd edn. London: UCL Press.

Department of Health (1991) Dietary Reference Values for Food Energy and Nutrients for the United Kingdom. COMA Report on Health and Social Subjects No. 41. London: HMSO.

Department of Health (1994) Nutritional Aspects of Cardiovascular Disease. Report on Health and Social Subjects No. 46. London: HMSO.

Department of Health (1995) Sensible Drinking: The report of an inter-department working group. London: HMSO.

Department of Health (1998) Nutritional Aspects of the Development of Cancer. Report on Health and Social Subjects No. 48. London: The Stationery Office.

Department of Health (2004) Choosing Health? Choosing a Better Diet. A consultation on priorities for a food and health action plan. London: The Stationery Office.

Food Standards Agency (2001) The Balance of Good Health. Information for educators and communicators. London: FSA

Health Education Authority (1996) Nutrition Briefing Paper. Scientific Basis of Nutrition Education: A synopsis of dietary reference values. London: HEA.

Health Education Authority, Department of Health and Ministry of Agriculture, Fisheries and Food (1994) The Balance of Good Health. London: HMSO.

Kromhout, D., Bosschieter, E.B. and Coulander, C.L. (1982) Dietary fibre and 10 year mortality from coronary heart disease, cancer and all causes. The Zutphen Study. Lancet ii: 508–521.

McCance, K.L. and Huether, S.E. (2002) Pathophysiology: The biologic basis for disease in adults and children, 4th edn. London: Mosby.

Marieb, E. (2004) Human Anatomy and Physiology, international edn. San Francisco, CA: Pearson Education.

Nursing and Midwifery Council (2002) Code of Professional Conduct. London: NMC.

Puska, P., Tuomilehto, J., Nissinen, A. and Vartiainen E. (eds) (1995) The North Kareliax Project: 20 Year Results and Experiences. Helsinki: Helsinki University Printing House.

Scientific Advisory Committee on Nutrition (SACN) (2004) Advice on Fish Consumption: Benefits and risks. London: TSO.

CHAPTER 7

Eating and drinking: nutrient and fluid replacement for health

JANE SAY

This chapter addresses particular nursing issues that arise in relation to eating and drinking within adult health care. It considers how to assess clients in relation to their nutritional and fluid needs and how to explore strategies that can be used to ensure that clients are receiving the most appropriate nutritional care. The key methods of replacing and maintaining fluid within the body are also explored.

Nutritional issues and clinical practice

Malnutrition

Within clinical practice clients will present with a number of nutritionally related problems and issues. Malnutrition is an overall term that can be defined as 'undernutrition due to inadequate food intake, dietary imbalance or nutrient deficiencies or overnutrition due to excess consumption' (McLaren 2003).

Obesity

Over the last 20 years the rates of obesity within the UK have doubled in children and tripled in adults (Sproston and Primatesta 2003). Currently two-thirds of the population in England and Wales are obese or overweight (House of Commons Health Committee 2004). Obesity can be defined as a body mass index (BMI) > 30 kg/m^2, whereas overweight can be defined as a BMI > 25 kg/m^2. (For a further discussion on BMI and its significance please see later.) Those defined as overweight or obese would normally have an excess of body fat stores.

If calorific intakes exceed energy expenditure (i.e. the total amount of energy used by the body to function metabolically, generate heat, synthesize new tissue and perform physical activity), the body will store increasing amounts of fat (as triglycerides) in the adipose tissue.

The reasons for the development of obesity are complex. Many social, personal and genetic factors are involved. However, within the UK two key factors related to our modern living have contributed to this epidemic: lack of physical activity and poor nutrition associated with excessive eating in the form of fast or junk foods.

Obesity is now seen as a major epidemic and can lead to complications such as Type 2 diabetes mellitus, heart disease and hypertension. The economic cost of the health problems caused by obesity has been estimated at £6.6–7.4 billion per year (House of Commons Health Committee 2004).

The government has now produced a document that aims to consider how society as a whole can tackle this issue (Department of Health [DoH] 2004). It hopes that individuals, communities, the NHS and other aspects of the public sector, local government, the voluntary and community sector, the food industry, employers and the media will all contribute to find reasonable solutions to this growing health problem. Nurses have a role to promote healthy eating and lifestyle choices in their clients.

Undernutrition

The problems associated with hospital undernutrition have been widely recognized for the last 25 years and a number of studies have identified the extent of undernutrition in hospital clients. Recent hospital figures suggest that this can range from 10% to 60% depending on the client population, the type of hospital and the criteria used to determine malnutrition (Hill et al. 1977, McWhirter and Pennington 1994, Naber et al. 1997, Strain et al. 1999, Vlaming et al. 1999, Watson 1999, Weekes 1999, Corish et al. 2000). This is also a problem for older adults in the community, and residents of long-stay institutions and nursing homes.

Malnutrition increases the risk of minor and major complications occurring; it extends the length of hospital stay and, as might be expected, increases the cost of treatment. Ultimately, for those patients who are malnourished the rate of morbidity and mortality is increased (Reilly et al. 1988, Sullivan et al. 1999). Extensive research on this area of care demonstrates that the maintenance of a client's nutritional status is vital in aiding recovery and rehabilitation (Veterans' Affairs' Total Parenteral Nutrition Study Group 1991).

The causes of undernutrition are complex but usually related to the disease process. However, other non-disease-related factors can also affect the client's nutritional status.

Disease-related factors

The nature of the disease can adversely affect appetite and this will lead to a reduction in food intake. Specific disabilities, which are associated with changes in mobility or sensation, can also affect how the client can eat and include:

• arthritis

- multiple sclerosis
- cerebrovascular accidents (or coma).

Such disabilities can also lead to a need for assistance during mealtimes. Physical factors such as poor oral hygiene/dentition, dysphagia and pain on eating can also influence nutritional intake. Changes in gastrointestinal tract function can have a very serious effect on food absorption and may cause nausea, vomiting and diarrhoea. In many illnesses there are changes in metabolic activity which can lead to increased requirements for protein and energy. Clients with severe burns or sepsis are known to have increased nutrient requirements. If such requirements are not met by the client's diet, deficiencies and undernutrition will occur. If the metabolic demands are very high the client can become undernourished very quickly. Any alterations in the client's psychological welfare, which includes conditions causing chronic pain and depression, can also affect appetite and nutritional intake. A number of treatments including multiple medication and aggressive drug therapies such as chemotherapy may also induce nutritional deficiencies (McLaren 2003).

Non-disease-related factors

Hospital/clinical routines and practices can also have a detrimental effect on clients' mealtimes. The Association of Community Health Councils (ACHC 1997) has identified a number of issues within clinical practice that affect clients' nutritional intakes:

- ordering and choice of food
- communication
- the quality and quantity of food
- positioning of clients and assistance with meals
- the eating environment
- the availability of utensils to assist those with physical disabilities.

The lack of nutritional assessment and monitoring has been highlighted by a number of authors (King's Fund 1992, Perry 1997, Maryon Davis and Bristow 1999). This lack means that those clients requiring help and support with nutrition are not identified or appropriately treated. Social and economic factors may also influence the way in which clients buy, choose and prepare their food, and if the appropriate support in the community is not available this may have a detrimental effect on their nutritional status.

Providing nutritional care in practice

Within clinical practice nutritional care is an essential element of nursing care. Recently, as part of the government's drive to improve the quality of client care, it has been identified as a 'fundamental aspect of care' that is 'crucial to the quality of a client's care experience' (DoH 2001a).

The Essence of Care

The Essence of Care (DoH 2001a) has identified food and nutrition as a fundamental aspect of care. For this it has produced a client-focused outcome statement that needs to be met in clinical practice. To aid health-care professionals in achieving this outcome it has identified 10 key factors that need to be addressed within practice. Each of these factors has a *benchmark* statement that describes best practice. These factors concentrate on the aspects of care such as assessment, assisting clients to eat and ensuring that the environment is conducive to eating.

Table 7.1 gives the client-focused outcome, and lists the factors needed to achieve this outcome along with their benchmark statements.

Table 7.1 Food and Nutrition Outcome and Benchmarking Statements

Agreed Patient/Client-Focused Outcome

Patients/clients are enabled to consume food (orally) which meets their individual need

	Factor	Benchmark of Best Practice
1	Screening/assessment to identify patients'/clients' nutritional needs	Nutritional screening progresses to **further assessment for all** patients/clients identified as **at risk**
2	Planning, implementation and evaluation of care for those patients who required a nutritional assessment	Plans of care based on **ongoing** nutritional assessments are devised, implemented and evaluated
3	A conducive environment (acceptable sights, sounds and smells)	The environment is **conducive** to enabling the **individual** clients to eat
4	Assistance with eating and drinking	Patients/clients **receive the care and assistance** they require with eating and drinking
5	Obtaining food	Patients/clients/carers, **whatever their communication needs**, are given sufficient information to enable them to obtain their food
6	Food provided	Food that is **provided by the service** meets the individual patients'/clients' needs
7	Food availability	Patients/clients who have set mealtimes are **offered a replacement meal if a meal is missed and can access snacks at any time**
8	Food presentation	Food is presented to patients/clients in a way that takes into account what **appeals to them as individuals**
9	Monitoring	The amount of food patients actually eat is **monitored and recorded**, and leads to **action** when it causes concern
10	Eating to promote health	**All opportunities** are used to encourage the patients/clients to eat to **promote** their own **health**

From *The Essence of Care* (DOH 2001a).

Screening/assessment to identify patients'/clients' nutritional needs

In many reports the requirement for all clients to receive nutritional screening or assessment on admission to hospital is viewed as vital if appropriate nutritional care is to be provided (King's Fund 1992, British Association of Parenteral and Enteral Nutrition [BAPEN] 1996, Maryon Davis and Bristow 1999, DoH 2001a, Royal College of Physicians 2002, Clinical Standards Board for Scotland 2002).

Nutritional screening is a relatively quick and simple method of identifying those clients who may be malnourished or 'at risk' of becoming malnourished while they are in hospital or receiving treatment. A follow-up and more in-depth assessment can then ensure that those clients who require and would most benefit from nutritional support are identified and appropriately treated. To continue monitoring of the client's nutritional status the screening should then be performed at weekly intervals. Unqualified staff, students, clients and carers may perform screening if they have received the necessary education and training and have been assessed as competent to use the screening tool. However, ultimate responsibility must lie with the registered practitioner (DoH 2001a). For clients who require a full nutritional assessment, a more detailed process is required. A registered practitioner who has the necessary education and training and has been assessed as competent must perform this. Within clinical practice this is likely to be a registered nurse (and may include a nutrition nurse specialist) or a dietitian.

To facilitate the screening process a number of screening tools have been developed that aim to determine the nutritional 'risk' status of the client (Royal College of Nursing [RCN] 1993, Reilly et al. 1995, Robshaw and Marbrow 1995, BAPEN 2003). These tools are based on factors that have been identified as significant in the development of malnutrition. An outline of these key factors is given in an adapted version of Reilly et al.'s (1995) nutrition risk score in Figure 7.1.

Body mass index

Measurement of the client's BMI is viewed as an important indicator of nutritional status. This measurement is determined from the weight and the height of the client and can be calculated as follows:

$$BMI = Weight (kg)/(Height \ in \ metres)^2.$$

The significance of the BMI measurement is given in Table 7.2.

This measurement closely correlates with body fat (Revicki and Israel 1986). However, it is important that the correct height (without shoes) and weight are obtained. In older people the measurement is less accurate

NUTRITION RISK SCORE CHART

Patient's name:

Hospital number: Ward:

Date: Time:

Weight: Height/Length: Signature:

Please circle relevant score. Only select one score from each section.
Select the highest score that applies.

		Score
1	ADULTS (> 18 years)	
	WEIGHT LOSS IN LAST 3 MONTHS (unintentional)	
	No weight loss	0
	0–3 kg weight loss	1
	> 3–6 kg weight loss	2
	6 kg or more	3
2	BMI (body mass index)	
	20 or more	0
	18 or 19	1
	15–17	2
	< 15	3
3	APPETITE	
	Good appetite, manages most of three meals/day (or equivalent)	0
	Poor appetite, poor intake – leaving more than half of meals provided (or equivalent)	2
	Appetite nil or virtually nil, unable to eat, NBM (for > four meals)	3
4	ABILITY TO EAT/RETAIN FOOD	
	No difficulties eating, able to eat independently No diarrhoea or vomiting	0
	Problems handling food, e.g. needs special cutlery Vomiting/frequent regurgitation (or possetting)/mild diarrhoea	1
	Difficulty swallowing, requiring modified consistency Problems with dentures, affecting food intake Problems with chewing, affecting food intake Slow to feed Moderate vomiting and/or diarrhoea (one to two/day for children) Needs help with feeding (e.g. physical handicap)	2
	Unable to take food orally. Unable to swallow (complete dysphagia) Severe vomiting and/or diarrhoea (more than two/day for children) Malabsorption	3

<pre>
5   STRESS FACTOR
       No stress factor (includes admission for investigation only)   0
       Mild   Minor surgery. Minor infection.   1
       Moderate   Chronic disease. Major surgery. Infections. Fractures   2
                         Pressure sores/ulcers. Cerebrovascular accident.
                         Inflammatory bowel disease
                         Other gastrointestinal disease
       Severe   Multiple injuries. Multiple fractures/burns. Multiple   3
                         deep pressure sores/ulcers. Severe sepsis.
                         Carcinoma/malignant disease
</pre>

                                                                    TOTAL:

DOCUMENTATION OF NUTRITION RISK SCORE

Date and time	Signature	Weight	Score	Comments

Action for nutritional risk assessment score

Complete on admission and then weekly for all patients.

Score	Risk status	Nutritional action plan
0–3	LOW	Check and record weight weekly. Monitor using nutrition risk score (NRS)
4–5	MEDIUM	Perform further assessment. Devise and implement a plan of care
6–15	HIGH	Perform further assessment. Devise and implement a plan of care and refer to the dietitian

Also refer to the Dietetic Department (via medical staff) if the patient needs specific advice about a special diet or education regarding a therapeutic diet.

Figure 7.1 Nutrition risk score chart. (Adapted from Reilly et al. 1995.)

Table 7.2 Body mass index (BMI) and its significance

BMI (kg/m^2)	Significance
< 18.5	Underweight, chronic undernutrition possible
18.5–20	Underweight, chronic undernutrition probable
20–25	Desirable weight, chronic malnutrition unlikely
25–30	Overweight, increased complications associated with chronic overnutrition
30–35	Moderately obese, increased complications associated with chronic overnutrition
35–40	Highly obese and at risk of complications associated with chronic overnutrition
> 40	Highly obese and at high risk of complications associated with chronic overnutrition

Adapted from Bowling (2004).

because it does not account for the loss of height and muscle mass that can occur in this group (Bowling 2004).

Weight loss

The percentage of recent weight loss is also viewed as an important method of determining nutritional status (Stiges-Serra and Franch-Arcas 1995). Based on the evidence available, the King's Fund (1992) stated that any client who has lost more than 10% of his or her body weight in the last 3 months should be offered nutritional support.

To determine weight loss over a 3- to 6-month period the following calculation is needed:

$$\text{Percentage weight loss} = \frac{\text{Usual weight in kg – Actual weight in kg}}{\text{Usual weight}} \times 100$$

If a client has ascites or oedema, allowances for the fluid weight must be made within the calculations. Often these clients will mask their true weight loss (Table 7.3).

Table 7.3 Masking of true weight loss

Percentage weight change over 3–6 months	Interpretation
< 5	Within normal variations
5–10	More than normal individual variation – early indicator of undernutrition risk
> 10	Clinically significant – requires nutritional support

Recent dietary intakes

The client's current and recent intakes should also be determined by questioning the client or his or her carer. Talking to the client about recent dietary intakes and how this may have changed requires the nurse to consider a range of issues relating to his or her everyday life. For each person, his or her circumstances and details will vary dramatically. However, it is important that the nurse can focus on the most relevant information and this should include details on the following:

- Any recent decrease in food intake.
- Changes in their appetite.
- Any difficulties with swallowing (also called dysphagia).
- Signs of recent weight loss, including clothes or rings becoming loose fitting.
- Any particular social or economic factors that may affect eating, including ability to afford the particular dietary requirements, ability to shop and prepare food, and any other support that the client requires to ensure adequate nutrition.
- The details of any psychological or physical disabilities that may have contributed to a change in nutritional status. This could include many different factors from poor dentition and a need for new dentures to chronic depression as a result of a severe illness.
- Any specialist dietary requirement. This may include a particular diet related to medical condition or may be specific to religious or cultural beliefs.

Stress factors/nature of current illness

During illness the nutritional requirements of the body can alter significantly. Metabolic activity can alter in response to the physical stress experienced by the body. This can mean that the resting energy requirements of the body may increase and, in clients with severe burns or sepsis, this can be as much as 60% (Kinney 1995). Many of the screening tools have a section that acknowledges the impact of specific illnesses on nutritional status and the scoring in the tool is weighted to demonstrate this. For some clients a specific deficiency may be found (such as iron deficiency anaemia). This may not lead to serious undernutrition, but the subsequent care and treatment that the client receives should reflect the increased requirements (such as for iron).

Further action, assessment and referral

The screening tools often include an action plan which details the steps to be taken next. For those clients who are identified as *high risk* or malnourished, the next step is usually referral to the dietitian and a more in-depth assessment is carried out. This assessment can then fully identify the specific nutritional care that the client is likely to require and may involve further referrals or the implementation of a specialist feeding regimen and an appropriate plan of care.

For those identified as *medium risk* or *at risk*, further assessment should be performed by a qualified practitioner and a care plan devised. Nutritional monitoring should continue on a weekly basis.

For those identified as *low risk*, the possibility of deterioration should be considered and these clients should be monitored on a regular basis. The timing of such monitoring will vary according to the nature of the client's condition and the type of care setting. The screening tool can also be used as a convenient means of monitoring.

Planning, implementation and evaluation of care for those patients who require a nutritional assessment

The Essence of Care (DoH 2001a) states that those clients who require further nutritional assessment should have a plan of care devised. This plan should be implemented and evaluated within the context of their ongoing nutritional assessment.

The details of the plan of care will obviously differ from client to client. However, it may involve a number of health-care professionals and include details of the specific nutritional support that is required by the client. The methods and timing of evaluation are also important if the care is to be properly monitored and its effectiveness assessed. Later a number of different methods of nutritional support and the associated care are addressed.

A conducive environment (acceptable sights, sounds and smells)

The environment in which clients eat can have a real effect on the whole experience of eating and drinking and can influence client intakes (ACHC 1997, Eberhardie 2000).

Food is more likely to be enjoyed if it is well cooked and presented and is of a good quality. Furthermore, if the client has particular requirements or follows a special diet (e.g. vegetarianism), then for him or her to like and appreciate the meal these issues must be acknowledged. Eating and drinking are normally sociable activities and the experience of a meal can be greatly improved if there is a social element to it.

In hospitals or residential care there may be very unpleasant sights, sounds and smells occurring during mealtimes. A client may be using a bedpan while others continue with their meal in the same room. The alarms on equipment in the area may be constantly ringing while nurses and doctors are busy dealing with a client in the next bed. Clients may not have been given the opportunity to wash their hands and the table and utensils may be dirty. All these factors will discourage clients from eating and can affect nutritional intakes.

Within a clinical area the registered nurse will have ultimate responsibility for the overall environment and organization of the area. However, unqualified staff, including health-care assistants, students, orderlies and housekeepers, may be given the responsibility, where it is thought appropriate, to carry out these activities. For all members of staff, the issues of ownership and accountability for this area of practice will need to be clear (DoH 2001a):

- Ensure that the environment is clean, including any tables, tablemats and cooking utensils.
- Wash your hands and remove dirty aprons before serving food.
- Give clients the opportunity to wash their hands.
- Where facilities allow, encourage eating at a communal table with other clients.
- Where possible encourage clients to eliminate before the meal begins.
- If a client requires the commode/toilet during mealtime take him or her to the bathroom.
- Ensure that the area is well ventilated to minimize bad odours and to remove old and stale cooking smells after the meal.
- Minimize unnecessary activity during mealtimes. If possible, introduce a dedicated mealtime approach where disruptions, visits, ward rounds and investigations are actively discouraged when the clients are eating.
- If the client wishes, encourage the involvement of their next of kin or carer during the mealtime period.

Assistance with eating and drinking

Many clients in hospital or residential care need extra assistance to eat their meals and, without such help, malnutrition can occur. This can be a particular issue with elderly clients and those with dementia. These groups of clients may have complex illnesses, previous malnutrition and increasing dependence (RCN 1993, McGillivray and Marland 1999). Clients themselves have commented on problems with appropriate positioning at mealtimes, lack of assistance with their meals and lack of appropriate utensils (ACHC 1997). In other work, clients have felt that nurses do not always recognize the impact of motor and physical disabilities on their eating behaviour (Sidenvall and Ek 1993).

As part of the initial screening and assessment process, those clients requiring extra help should be clearly identified. For some clients, simple strategies may be sufficient to ensure that they can manage to feed themselves. This may include the provision of special crockery or cutlery. Other clients may need one-to-one assistance at each mealtime, and without such assistance they would not be able to eat. For all clients independence should be promoted. This may be achieved through further education of clients and their carers. The involvement of other members of the multidisciplinary team (MDT) may also be required, particularly if specialist equipment is needed. Clients who have difficulty swallowing should be referred to a speech and language therapist for further treatment. Some of the key actions that will assist clients in their eating and drinking include:

- Where possible sit or support the client in an upright chair with easy access to the table and food.
- Clients in bed should be sitting/supported upright with easy access to their table and food.
- Ensure that those clients who need dentures have them.
- Ensure that the mouth is clean.
- Assess for pain or nausea well before mealtimes so that appropriate action can be taken in time for the meal.
- Ensure that the appropriate member of staff gives any particular drug therapies due before mealtimes (e.g. insulin therapy).
- Ensure that any specialist utensils, fresh water, a hot drink and condiments are available.
- Ensure that clients receive the meal of their choice which is suitable for their specialist dietary, religious or cultural requirements.
- Be sensitive to clients' needs and any embarrassment they may have about eating.
- Where necessary, protect the client's clothes with a napkin.
- Help the client with difficult packaging and rearrange the tray/plate to ensure that he or she can reach its contents.
- Ensure that hot food or drinks are not likely to spill and injure the client.
- Explain to those clients who are confused or disoriented that it is mealtime.
- When helping a client to eat, sit at the same level so that you can reach him or her comfortably and make eye contact.
- Communicate with your client as you feed him or her.
- Give half to one teaspoonful per mouthful and place on the stronger side of the mouth if the client has hemiplegia (paralysis on one side of the body) or hemiparesis (weakness on one side of the body).
- Allow the client time to chew and swallow twice before giving the next mouthful.
- Ask the client to clear the throat between each mouthful to ensure that the airway is clear.
- Ask the client to cough during and at the end of the meal. This will also clear the airway.
- If the client shows any signs of distress, uncontrolled coughing or has a gurgly sounding voice, STOP FEEDING IMMEDIATELY and seek qualified assistance. This could be a sign of aspiration (food entering the respiratory tract).
- At the end of the meal, check the mouth for retained food and offer a drink or a mouthwash where necessary.
- To aid digestion, allow the client to remain upright for at least half an hour after the meal.
- For those patients who require regular assistance, try to ensure that the

same personnel are involved. If the client agrees, and where appropriate, encourage the next of kin or carer to help with feeding.

It is important that staff have been appropriately trained in providing this care and that they recognize their roles and responsibilities in carrying out these activities.

Obtaining food, food provided, food availability and food presentation

Within *The NHS Plan* (DoH 2000), a clear commitment was made by the government to improve hospital food. To further this commitment the *Better Hospital Food Programme* (DoH 2001b) was launched. This programme detailed specific actions that hospitals and NHS trusts needed to perform in order to improve food provision. The focus of this work was principally on the nature of hospital/NHS catering services and included issues such as menu design, the nature and type of hospital food, food preparation and delivery, and the overall catering service. Many of the issues identified relate to the factors within *The Essence of Care* (DoH 2001a).

The need for improvements in the quality and nutritional content of hospital food, alongside a more comprehensive catering service, has been recognized for some time (ACHC 1997, Bond 1997, Maryon Davis and Bristow 1999). In response to previous reports, the *Better Hospital Food Programme* (DoH 2001b) has initiated the introduction of a minimum standard for hospital meals. This will consist of breakfast, light lunch, two-course evening dinner, drinks and snacks on at least two occasions and the provision of a 24-hour catering service. This round-the-clock service comprises three elements: the ward kitchen service, the snack box and the light bite.

For more information on this programme visit the NHS Estates website at: http://patientexperience.nhsestates.gov.uk/bhf/bhf_content/home/home.asp

Below are some key activities that are needed to ensure that clients receive the most appropriate menu choice:

- Ensure that clients and carers understand the nature of the menu, and how to complete it.
- Particular requirements (medical, cultural and religious), and how they can be met, should be discussed with clients and carers.
- On admission, inform catering and the dietitian of specialist dietary requirements. (The previous two points may well form part of the initial screening/assessment process for which a registered nurse or clearly identified health-care professional should be responsible.)
- An identified person should assist clients who have difficulty completing their menu choices.
- Regular staff should be designated to serve food and drinks to clients.

- While serving meals ward staff should check that clients are receiving the correct meal at the right temperature.
- Clients who miss a meal should be offered a suitable alternative via the 24-hour service that is available.
- Preparation of food and food storage in the area (including the client's own food) must follow health and hygiene standards.

Completing menus and serving food may be designated to a number of unqualified staff within the ward team (including health-care assistants, orderlies and housekeepers). However, it is important that staff have been appropriately trained in providing this care and that they recognize their roles and responsibilities in carrying out these activities.

Monitoring

The need for continued nutritional monitoring of clients during hospital stays has also been recognized as necessary to ensure a client's nutritional care (RCN 1993, ACHC 1997, Bond 1997). It is important to monitor the nutritional intake of clients and to re-screen or re-assess them throughout their stay. Normally re-screening or re-assessment would be performed on a weekly basis; monitoring food intake needs to be performed and action taken if there is any cause for concern (DoH 2001a). Previous work has found that there may be lack of documentation of nutritional care and no clear strategy for nutritional care (including monitoring) (Perry 1997).

Eating to promote their own health

In Chapter 6 the components of a healthy diet were discussed alongside simple recommendations on how to achieve such a diet by following *The Balance of Good Health* (HEA et al. 1994, Food Standards Agency [FSA] 2001) guidelines; this chapter should be revisited.

The guidelines in *The Balance of Good Health* are for healthy members of the population. Within clinical practice, following screening or assessment registered practitioners, including nurses, dietitians and doctors, will determine whether the guidelines in *The Balance of Good Health* are appropriate or whether they need to educate the client about more specialized diets.

For those who can follow the guidelines, it is important that nurses support and advise clients on achieving them. This will also include the next of kin and carers who may be the main people to do the shopping and cooking. As with other aspects of nutritional care, it is important that the staff involved in promoting healthy eating are properly trained. Within the clinical area the availability of displays, handouts and leaflets will also facilitate the promotion of healthy eating.

The following websites offer straightforward advice on how to achieve a healthy diet. They also have material that can be downloaded to support this advice.

- Food Standards Agency: www.foodstandards.gov.uk/aboutus/ publications/
- British Nutrition Foundation: www.nutrition.org.uk
- Weight Wise (Developed by the British Dietetic Association): www. bdaweightwise.com

Nutritional support

Oral feeding is always the preferred method of meeting a client's nutritional needs. However, for some clients it will not be possible to follow a normal healthy diet and extra nutritional support may be necessary. Initially, a full nutritional assessment of the client will be needed and the dietitian will then determine the most appropriate method of nutritional support.

In practice the nurses, dietitians and medical team will all consider the most appropriate form of feeding. Figure 7.2 provides an aid for this decision-making process.

Improving oral intakes

Changes in the hospital menu, along with the availability of food and how it is presented and served, are all aimed at improving patients' oral intakes (DoH 2001a, 2001b). Food can be supplemented or fortified by adding cream or cheese. This increases the protein and energy content of the food. It is important for nurses to ensure that (if appropriate) clients choose and receive high-protein/high-energy meals and are given extra high-energy/high-protein snacks.

Oral supplements

These should be used for clients who cannot maintain their nutritional intakes from everyday food and drink. Although supplements have been proved to have real benefits (Delmi et al. 1990), it is important that they are used appropriately because they are often wasted. There are a number of supplements available in liquid, semi-solid or powder form. Some are nutritionally complete whereas others will only 'supplement' the usual oral diet. A dietitian would normally assess the need for supplements and decide the most appropriate supplement for the client. Within the clinical setting it is part of the nurse's role to ensure that clients receive and take the supplement. This activity should be monitored and recorded so that a proper evaluation can be performed. Unqualified staff may be supervised by registered nurses to help with this activity.

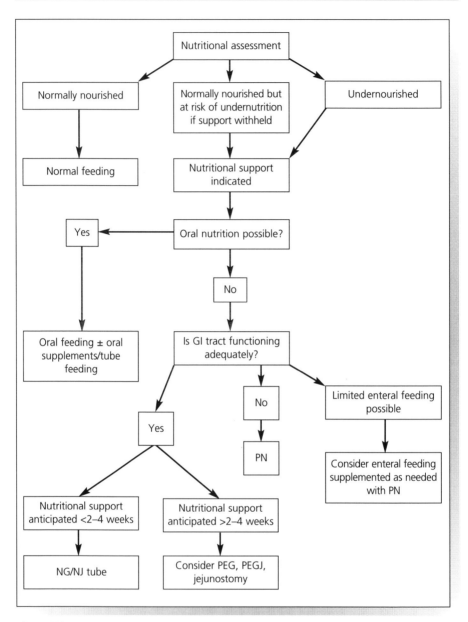

Figure 7.2
Choices for nutritional support: a
decision-making process. GI,
gastrointestinal; NG, nasogastric; NJ,
nasojejunal; PEG, percutaneous
endoscopically placed gastrostomy; PEGJ,
percutaneous endoscopically placed
gastro-jejunostomy; PN, parenteral
nutrition. (Adapted from Bowling 2004.)

Enteral (or tube) feeding

This method of feeding delivers a liquid feed via a tube directly into the gastrointestinal tract. Clients can receive all their nutritional needs in this way or it may be used as a means of supplementing oral intakes. The type of feed used will depend on the clients' requirements, their current dietary intake, the function of their gastrointestinal tracts and their clinical condition (certain conditions such as liver and renal disease may require a specialized diet).

Clients (and their carers) who are receiving nutritional support in this way may be anxious and may need reassurance and explanations about the treatment involved. Always refer any questions from the client or the carers to the appropriate member of staff. Receiving a tube feed can reduce the pleasurable aspects of eating; as such the client may need psychological and social support while receiving this type of feed.

Another aspect of care that must be given attention is the client's oral hygiene or mouth care. Some clients will be nil by mouth (NBM) and this may cause problems in the mouth such as dryness, cracking, stomatitis (inflammation of the mouth), pain, ulcers and infection. Therefore clients undergoing tube feeding need a careful assessment of their oral hygiene needs, and the specific care required for preventing oral complications needs to be highlighted. There are three methods of enteral feeding:

1. Nasogastric (NG) feeding: a tube is passed via the nasopharynx into the stomach.
2. Nasojejunal (NJ) feeding: a tube is passed via the nasopharynx and stomach and on into the jejunum.
3. Percutaneous endoscopically placed gastrostomy or jejunostomy (PEG/ PEJ) feeding: a tube is inserted directly into the stomach or jejunum via the abdominal wall.

Table 7.4 gives a summary of the main considerations for these types of feed.

Specific nursing care associated with enteral feeding

Nasogastric feeding/nasojejunal feeding

NG tube insertion/ensuring the correct position

- NG tube insertion: this is normally performed by either a registered nurse or qualified doctor. Within the clinical area local policies and guidelines should be used to advise on the exact procedures for insertion and checking of the tube position.

Table 7.4 The types of enteral feed and their specific considerations

Type of feed	Indications	Contraindications	Practical considerations
NG	Short-term use for clients with use of stomach and no vomiting or aspiration Also impaired swallowing (e.g. stroke), altered consciousness, ventilated clients, dysphagia For supplementation of inadequate oral intakes Psychological requirements, e.g. anorexia nervosa	Obstruction preventing passage of tube Impaired stomach emptying caused by obstruction Intestinal obstruction Intestinal perforation or nearby gastrointestinal fistula Severe facial injury	Two main types of tubes may be used: fine bore or wide bore (e.g. Ryles). Normally a fine-bore tube is used Care of the NG tube, including: Passing the tube Ensuring correct position Regular checking of tube position Feed administration Complications, including removal by the patient; this may be as a result of confusion or on purpose as a means of withdrawing consent. Ulceration/narrowing/strictures of the oesophagus. This is unusual when fine-bore tubes are used. Diarrhoea
NJ	Short-term use for clients whose stomach needs to be bypassed and where there is no vomiting In clients with a high risk of aspiration Pancreatitis	As per NG feeding – see above	Two main types of tube may be used: single lumen (can be placed with or without an endoscope) or double lumen (needs specialist placement) Care of the NJ tube, including: Passing the tube (normally done endoscopically) Ensuring correct position (normally done under radiology) Regular checking of tube position Feed administration Complications as per NG feeding – see above
PEG/PEJ	For longer-term feeding > 4 weeks Used particularly in cerebrovascular accidents (stroke), head injury, multiple sclerosis, motor neuron disease, severe physical and learning disabilities	Ascites, severe obesity, blood clotting abnormalities, oesophageal or gastric varices (varicose veins in the gastrointestinal tract), gastric ulceration or malignancy	Care of the PEG/PEJ tube, including: Insertion of the tube (performed endoscopically by medical personnel) Checking and management of insertion site Feed administration Complications: peritonitis, aspiration, infection of the site, haemorrhage, tube blockage, death of tissue (necrosis) around the site caused by pressure from the tube limiting the local blood supply

NG, nasogastric; NJ, nasojejunal; PEG, percutaneous endoscopically placed gastrostomy; PEJ, percutaneous endoscopically placed jejunostomy.

- NG tube position: this should be done at the following times (Bowling 2004): on initial placement, before a feed, before giving medication (if the tube is not being used), following vomiting or coughing, after tube dislodgement and if the patient complains of discomfort.

For a comprehensive step-by-step account of how to insert and check an NG tube, please refer to local policies and procedures.

NJ tube insertion/ensuring the correct position

- NJ tube insertion: this is normally performed by medical staff using endoscopy and can be checked using radiographs.
- NJ tube position: to avoid displacement of the tube it must be securely fixed to the nose or cheek. A permanent mark should be made at the point where the tube leaves the nose. The position should be checked before starting a feed. If there are signs that the tube may have moved report this to the appropriate registered practitioner (registered nurse, dietitian, doctor or nutritional nurse specialist). **Do not** start a feed until the position is confirmed.

NG/NJ feed administration

A registered nurse will have ultimate responsibility for the management of the feed. However, unqualified staff may provide aspects of care after receiving the appropriate training.

The guidelines below outline how to deliver an NG or NJ feed and have been adapted from Bowling (2004), but always refer to local policies and procedures when delivering this type of care:

- Before any feed starts, the position of the tube must be checked according to local policy and procedures (see above). **Do not** start a feed until the position of the tube is confirmed. Remember that there is a significant risk of pulmonary aspiration (feed entering the lungs) if the tube is misplaced.
- Wash hands thoroughly and use a clean apron before beginning the procedure. Hygiene is extremely important when dealing with these feeds. NJ feeds carry a greater risk of infection because the acid environment of the stomach is bypassed and this would normally act as a barrier to infection.
- Position clients at a 30–45° upright angle unless their medical condition does not allow this (e.g. spinal injury). Keep upright for 1 hour after the feed to avoid aspiration as a result of reflux.
- For NG feeding, two methods of feeding may be used: pump feeding, where an infusion pump continuously delivers the feed at a rate of about 100 ml/h (this is determined by the dietitian), or gravity feeding, where a 50- to 60-ml syringe containing feed is attached to the giving set. This is held higher than the client and is allowed to drain into the NG tube.

- For NJ feeding, a pump feed will be used. The initial rate will be slower because the small intestine cannot hold as much fluid and it will be increased slowly over time.
- Feeding duration will vary according to the method of delivery and the requirements of the client. Normally, a break in feeding is given to clients on NG feeds. However, NJ feeds can continue over the full 24 hours.
- Administer the feed as prescribed and documented by the dietitian. Ensure that the correct feed is given at the correct time and rate of delivery.
- To prevent blockage the NG tube should be flushed with 50 ml cooled boiled (at home) or sterile (in the acute setting) water before and after feeds and medication. The NJ tube should be flushed every 6 h with 30 ml sterile water using a 50-ml syringe.
- Record the amount of feed given.
- Report and record any complications immediately.
- Continue nutritional monitoring and screening to help evaluate the effectiveness of the feeding regimen.

Percutaneous endoscopically placed gastrostomy or jejunostomy

PEG/PEJ feeding

This type of feeding is used with clients who require enteral feeding for more than 4 weeks. The tube requires surgical placement using endoscopy. As with the other types of enteral feeding, the responsibility for the client's care will remain with the registered nurse; unqualified staff who have been properly trained may be involved with some aspects of care.

Care after a PEG/PEJ insertion

Initial care after insertion is based on monitoring the client's physiological status following an invasive surgical procedure. Any changes in the client's condition can then be quickly acted upon and further complications prevented:

- After the procedure, monitor and record temperature, pulse, respirations and blood pressure every half hour for 4 hours, then every hour for 2 hours. Report any changes in the client's observations immediately to the registered nurse.
- Report any signs or complaints of pain to the registered nurse. Analgesia can then be given.
- The client will remain NBM and nil by tube for 6 h after the procedure.
- Inspect the insertion site for blood or serous fluid leakage. Immediately report any leakage or continuous bleeding to a registered nurse or doctor because further dressing or suturing may be required.

- After 6 h the tube may be flushed with sterile water.
- The dietitian will determine the full feeding regimen (course of treatment).

PEG/PEJ feed administration

The principles of care related to this type of feeding are similar to those of NG and NJ feeding. However, particular care of the insertion site is needed to prevent infection. If the site requires cleaning, full aseptic technique must be used. After 5–6 weeks (when a fibrous tract develops through the abdominal wall), the original tube may be removed and a more compact skin level gastrostomy 'button' tube is inserted. This offers a neat, easily managed tube for longer-term feeding. When this type of feeding is no longer needed the tube is removed via endoscopy. The ongoing care of PEG and PEJ feeding is more specialized than NG and NJ feeding. To examine these in more depth please refer to local policies and procedures.

Parenteral nutrition

Parenteral nutrition (PN) is a very specialized and invasive method of feeding. It is the administration of nutrient solutions via a central or peripheral vein. Several members of the MDT including registered nurses, doctors, dietitians and pharmacists manage this type of feeding. It is normally used with clients whose gastrointestinal tract is not working or not accessible. To carry out this type of feed, a dedicated feeding line is established. To do this a catheter is passed either centrally (via the subclavian or jugular veins) or peripherally (via the basilar or cephalic veins of the arm). The pharmacy then prepares the sterile infusion of nutrients, based on the particular nutrient requirements of the client as determined by the dietitian and medical team. The care for this type of feed is highly specialized and beyond the remit of this chapter

Fluid management in clinical practice

Within clinical practice the maintenance of a client's hydration is a fundamental aspect of care. Many clients will be able to maintain an appropriate fluid balance that ensures health. For those who are eating and drinking normally there may be little concern. However, changes in a client's condition or particular clinical interventions may alter his or her ability to maintain fluid balance. Overall there are three main causes of fluid imbalance:

1. Excessive losses, e.g. vomiting and diarrhoea.
2. Reduced intake, e.g. loss of thirst mechanism which can occur in altered levels of consciousness/confused states; lack of access to water which can occur in clients who are bed bound or again in those with altered levels of

consciousness/confused states; and inappropriate/inadequate intake resulting from improper intravenous fluid regimens. Both excessive losses and reduced intakes will lead to a client becoming dehydrated.
3. Fluid retention, e.g. in heart or kidney failure, and excessive fluid replacement can lead to fluid overload where the body has an excess of fluids.

To determine any potential or actual fluid imbalance it is important first to assess the client's fluid status.

Clinical assessment of fluid balance

A history of the client's recent fluid input and output along with any particular difficulties related to their fluid balance need to be obtained. This must recognize planned and future interventions that will affect intakes, e.g. when a client is NBM for surgery. They may not be able to eat and drink normally after treatments such as chemotherapy or extensive head and neck surgery. The monitoring of fluid input and output alongside laboratory findings is vital, and even weight can be used to assess a client's fluid balance.

Table 7.5 summarizes the key means of determining a client's fluid status.

Fluid input and output charts

This is a common means of monitoring fluid balance and can act as an important part of the assessment and monitoring process.

How a fluid balance chart should be maintained

- The registered nurse or other registered practitioner will determine the need for a fluid balance chart. All clients receiving intravenous fluids should be given a fluid balance chart.
- Inform the client, the carers and all other staff involved in the care about the fluid balance chart.
- Measure intake from all sources, i.e. oral fluids, intravenous fluids, enteral feeds (including water used to flush the tube), fluid medication, liquid food (e.g. soup).
- Accurately measure output from all sources, i.e. urine output (either bedpan, urinal or catheter), NG drainage, drainage tubes, diarrhoea, wound drainage and vomit.
- Record input and output on the chart.
- At the end of each 24-hour period, total the client's input and output values. Higher input values than output values indicate a positive fluid balance, whereas lower input values than output values indicate a negative fluid balance.
- Weigh the patient daily at the same time and in the same clothes. Sudden and acute weight changes are indicative of fluid gains/losses. Remember that 1 litre of water weighs 1 kg. These changes can then be assessed against the fluid balance record from each day.

Table 7.5 Assessment of fluid status

Observation	Fluid excess	Dehydration
History of recent fluid balance[a]	Reduced urine output (oliguria) No urine output (anuria) Excessive urine output (polyuria)	Reduced urine output (oliguria) No urine output (anuria) Excessive urine output (polyuria) Diarrhoea Vomiting Polydipsia (excessive thirst) Excessive faecal fistula losses Unable to eat or drink normally
	Note that oliguria/anuria can occur in conditions such as renal failure and will cause an excess of fluid in the body	Note that oliguria/anuria will normally occur in dehydrated clients. However, conditions such as diabetes mellitus can lead to polyuria and cause dehydration if intake is not maintained
		A faecal fistula can occur when a tract develops from the bowel to the abdominal surface, where it oozes faecal fluid. This may occur after bowel surgery or in certain cancers
Physical assessment[a]	Firm, protruding eyeballs Oedema Ascites Bounding pulse Taut shiny skin	Eyeballs sunken Dry and flaky skin Dry cracked mouth Weak, thready pulse
Vital signs[b]		
Blood pressure	Increased	Decreased (especially on standing)
Pulse	Increased	Increased
Temperature	Unchanged	Elevated
Respirations	Increased rate	Unchanged or increased
Key laboratory findings[b]		
Urine specific gravity	Decreased (around 1.003)	Increased (around 1.025 or more)
Serum sodium	< 135 mmol/l	> 145 mmol/l

Cont.

Table 7.5 *Cont.*

Observation	Fluid excess	Dehydration
Hourly urine output[b]	> 60 ml/h (note that normally hydrated individuals can have an output > 60 ml/h)	< 30–50 ml/h (note that this may not be the case if the client has polyuria caused by diabetes mellitus)
Weight[b]: this must be assessed in the context of a client's nutritional status. Acute losses and increases (over hours/a few days) are usually associated with fluid movement	A 5% gain	A loss of 2–6% may indicate dehydration

[a]These observations are based on a subjective or personal view of the client's presentation and as such may not always be accurate.
[b]These observations are based on more objective measurements and offer a more accurate means of determining fluid status.

- Significant changes in the client's input and output need to be reported to the registered nurse and doctor in case further monitoring or intervention is required.

Urine output that falls below 30 ml/h over 2 consecutive hours can be indicative of renal failure, internal bleeding or dehydration. Further investigations and treatment would be urgently started if this occurs.

Maintaining fluid intakes

The daily fluid balance in adults normally comprises an input of 2400 ml and an output of 2400 ml; this can vary from day to day.

Oral intakes

Below are some of the key issues that have been previously raised. They incorporate aspects from *The NHS Plan* (DoH 2000), *The Essence of Care* document (DoH 2001a) and the *Better Hospital Food Programme* (DoH 2001b):

- Those clients requiring help with eating and drinking need to be identified and the appropriate assistance given.
- Where possible sit the client up in a comfortable position.
- If appropriate, encourage carers to help clients to drink and bring in extra drinks that the client enjoys (within any specialist dietary or fluid restrictions).

- Those dedicated to providing meals should also be involved in aiding the client to drink.
- Ensure that specialist utensils are provided to help the client to drink normally.
- In hospital more than seven beverages should be offered each day along with fresh drinking water (DoH 2000).
- Throughout the day offer fluids on a regular basis.
- If needed record and document all fluid intakes accurately.

Intravenous therapy

For some clients it will not be possible to maintain an adequate oral intake. In this case intravenous therapy will be an important means of ensuring adequate fluid intakes. The choice of fluid will be determined by the client's condition and prescribed by the doctor. There are a variety of intravenous fluids that are used to maintain electrolyte and fluid balance. Physiological (0.9% or normal) saline contains water and the electrolytes sodium and chloride. In this solution there is specifically 0.9 g sodium chloride per 100 ml water. Other solutions contain glucose and water only (sometimes called a dextrose solution since dextrose is another term for glucose). A 5% glucose solution contains 5 g glucose in 100 ml water. There are also other forms of intravenous fluids that have combinations of glucose and saline and some that contain sodium lactate or sodium bicarbonate. The choice and amount of intravenous fluids for fluid replacement are very dependent on the patient's condition and will be influenced by their blood results.

There are specific management issues related to intravenous infusions that are beyond the scope of this chapter.

Conclusion

This chapter has demonstrated how to maintain adequately a client's eating and drinking while they are in our care. The importance of nutritional and fluid assessment and screening has been addressed. The specific components that need to be considered when carrying out such assessments have also been discussed. A wide range of interventions has been considered to ensure that clients receive the most appropriate nutritional and fluid balance care. The need for a healthy approach to dietary intakes has been examined in the light of increasing rates of obesity and nutritionally related disease processes. Finally, the issues raised within this chapter have been placed in the context of the current changes within the NHS as a result of *The NHS Plan* (DoH 2000).

References

Association of Community Health Councils (1997) Health News Briefing. Hungry in hospital. London: ACHC.

Bond, S. (ed.) (1997) Eating matters: A resource for improving dietary care in hospitals. Centre for Health Services Research, University of Newcastle upon Tyne.

Bowling, T. (ed.) (2004) Nutritional Support for Adults and Children: A handbook for hospital practice. Oxford: Radcliffe Medical Press.

British Association of Parenteral and Enteral Nutrition (1996) Standards and Guidelines for Nutritional Support of Patients in Hospitals. Maidenhead: BAPEN.

British Association of Parenteral and Enteral Nutrition (2003) Screening Tool for Adults at Risk of Malnutrition. Maidenhead: BAPEN.

Clinical Standards Board for Scotland (2002) Draft Clinical Standards. Food, fluid and nutritional care. Edinburgh: CSBS.

Corish, C.A., Flood, P., Mulligan, S. and Kennedy, N.P. (2000) Apparent low frequency of undernutrition in Dublin hospitals' in-patients: should we review the anthropometric thresholds for clinical practice? British Journal of Nutrition 84: 325–355.

Delmi, M., Rapin, C.H., Bengoa, J.M., Delmas, P.D., Vasey, P. and Bonjour, J.P. (1990) Dietary supplementation in elderly patients with fractured neck of femur. The Lancet 335: 1013–1016.

Department of Health (2000) The NHS Plan. London: HMSO.

Department of Health (2001a) The Essence of Care. Patient focussed benchmarking for health professionals. London: HMSO.

Department of Health (2001b) Better Hospital Food Programme. Press release 21/9/01. London: DoH.

Department of Health (2004) Choosing Health? Choosing a Better Diet. A consultation on priorities for a food and health action plan. London: The Stationery Office.

Eberhardie, C. (2000) Practical Eating and Feeding Skills. NT Clinical Monograph. London: Nursing Times Books.

Food Standards Agency (2001) The Balance of Good Health. Information for Educators and Communicators. London: FSA.

Health Education Authority, Department of Health and Ministry of Agriculture, Fisheries and Food (1994) The Balance of Good Health. London: HMSO.

Hill, G.L., Blackett, R.L., Pickerford, I. et al. (1977) Malnutrition in surgical patients – an unrecognised problem. Lancet i: 689.

House of Commons Health Committee (2004) Obesity, Vol. 1. HCP 23-I. Third Report of session 2003–04. London: The Stationery Office.

King's Fund (1992) A Positive Approach to Nutrition as Treatment: A report of the Working Party chaired by Lennard-Jones on the role of enteral and parenteral feeding in hospital and at home. London: King's Fund.

Kinney, J.M. (1995) Metabolic response to starvation, injury and sepsis. In: Payne-James, J., Grimble, G. and Silk, D. (eds), Artificial Nutrition Support in Clinical Practice. London: Edward Arnold, pp. 1–11.

McGillivray, T. and Marland, G. (1999) Assisting demented patients with feeding: problems in a ward environment. A review of the literature. Journal of Advanced Nursing 29: 608–614.

McLaren, S. (2003) Disease related malnutrition. In: The Nursing Times: Nutrition, a practical guide. London: Emap.

McWhirter, J.P. and Pennington, C.R. (1994) Incidence and recognition of malnutrition in hospital. British Medical Journal 308: 945–948.

Maryon Davis, A. and Bristow, A. (1999) Managing Nutrition in Hospital: A recipe for quality. London: The Nuffield Trust.

Naber, T.H.J., de Bree, A., Schermer, T.R.J., Bakkeren, J., Bar, B., de Wild, G. and Katan, M.B. (1997) Specificity of indexes and malnutrition when applied to apparently healthy people: the effect of age. American Journal of Clinical Nutrition 65: 1721–1725.

Perry, L. (1997) Nutrition a hard nut to crack. An exploration of the knowledge, attitudes and activities of qualified nurses in relation to nutritional nursing care. Journal of Clinical Nursing 6: 315–324.

Reilly, J.J., Hull, S.F., Albert, N., Waller, A. and Bringardener, S. (1988) Economic impact of malnutrition: a model system for hospitalised patients. Journal of Parenteral and Enteral Nutrition 12: 371–376.

Reilly, H.M., Martineau, J.K., Moran, A. and Kennedy, H. (1995) Nutritional screening – evaluation and implementation of a simple nutrition risk score. Clinical Nutrition 14: 269–273.

Revicki, D.A. and Israel, R.G. (1986) Relationship between body mass indices and measure of body adiposity. American Journal of Public Health 76: 992–994.

Robshaw, V. and Marbrow, S. (1995) Raising awareness of patients' nutritional state. Professional Nurse 111: 41–42.

Royal College of Nursing (1993) Nutrition Standards and the Older Adult. RCN Dynamic Quality Improvement Programme. London: RCN.

Royal College of Physicians (2002) Nutrition and Patients. A Doctor's Responsibility. Report of a Working Party of the Royal College of Physicians. London: RCP.

Sidenvall, B. and Ek, A.C. (1993) Long term care patients and their dietary intake related to eating ability and nutritional needs: nursing staff interventions. Journal of Advanced Nursing 18: 565–573.

Sproston, K. and Primatesta, P. (2003) Health Survey for England 2002. London: The Stationery Office.

Stiges-Serra, A. and Franch-Arcas, G.E. (1995) Nutrition assessment. In: Payne-James, J., Grimble, G. and Silk, D. (eds), Artificial Nutrition Support in Clinical Practice. London: Edward Arnold.

Strain, N.C., Wright, C.E., Ward, K. and Shaffer, J.L. (1999) Can the true prevalence of malnutrition be assessed at admission to hospital? Proceedings of the Nutrition Society 58: 112A.

Sullivan, D.H., Sun, S. and Walls, R.C. (1999) Protein energy undernutrition among elderly hospitalised patients. Journal of the American Medical Association 281: 2013–2019.

Veterans' Affairs' Total Parenteral Nutrition Study Group (1991) Perioperative total parenteral nutrition in surgical patients. New England Journal of Medicine 325: 525–532.

Vlaming, S., Biehler, A., Chattopadhyay, S., Jamieson, C., Cunliffe, A. and Powell-Tuck, J. (1999) Nutritional status of patients on admission to acute services of a London teaching hospital. Proceedings of the Nutrition Society 58: 119A.

Watson, J.L. (1999) The prevalence of malnutrition in patients admitted to care of the elderly wards. Proceedings of the Nutrition Society 58: 139A.

Weekes, E. (1999) The incidence of malnutrition in medical patients admitted to a hospital in south London. Proceedings of the Nutrition Society 58: 126A.

CHAPTER 8

Elimination: alimentary and urinary tracts

M. NAIR

Few of us give serious thought to our digestive system until something goes wrong. Often, little attention is given to what we eat, how the food eaten is broken down, how the nutrients are absorbed and finally how the digestive system is emptied. The government and the media frequently promote healthy eating in order to ensure that our digestive systems are in good working order.

The alimentary tract is also known as the digestive system or the gastrointestinal tract. It involves the mouth, pharynx, oesophagus, stomach and intestines. The main function of the alimentary tract is to provide nutrients, water and electrolytes for the body. These are obtained from food eaten and fluids drunk; to carry out this function the gastrointestinal tract performs the roles of digestion, absorption and the elimination of unwanted materials (Figure 8.1).

The breakdown of food, making it soluble, is called digestion (Clancy and McVicar 1995). This involves two processes: mechanical and chemical. Mechanical processes break down large pieces of food into smaller food substances, whereas chemical processes break the food into simpler substances. These soluble substances are then absorbed to provide nutrients for the cells of the body's tissues. Any undigested food, water, bacteria and dead cells of the lining of the digestive tract are eliminated.

The alimentary tract is a continuous tract and is approximately 10 m long from the mouth to the anus. The small intestine is around 6 m long and the large intestine is in the region of 1.5 m long (Mader 1997). The accessory organs of digestion lie outside the tract and secrete various chemicals that aid digestion. The accessory organs are the salivary glands, liver, pancreas and gallbladder. They produce various enzymes that help break down foodstuffs, e.g. salivary amylase (ptyalin) will act on sugars and starch in the diet whereas pepsin will act on proteins. Other accessory organs include the lips, teeth, tongue and palate.

This chapter is concerned with a brief anatomy and physiology of the gastrointestinal tract, some of the common problems associated with this system and the nursing management related to this.

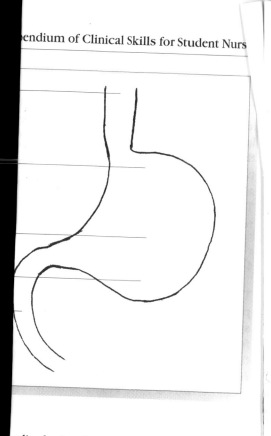

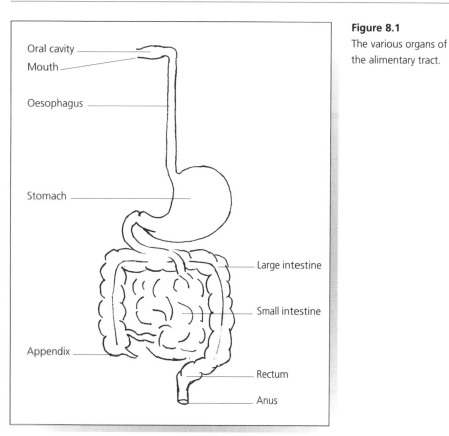

Figure 8.1
The various organs of the alimentary tract.

udinal, circular and oblique muscles. This
ysical action.
igestive enzymes also help to break down
gestion. During chemical digestion, semi-
nto a semi-liquid form. Enzymes such as
vert them to peptones; gastric lipase will
converts the soluble protein of milk into

stomach

n and mixed with HCl
ones
e
omach
num via the pylorus
amin B_{12} is formed in the stomach.

ameter compared with that of the large
ic sphincter to the ileocaecal valve of the
ngth.

The oral cavity

Mouth

The mouth is the start of the alimentary canal. It receives food and the mechanical breakdown of food particles begins here. The broken down food particles are mixed with saliva (Shier et al. 2004). The activity of breaking down foodstuff and mixing it with saliva is called mastication. This broken-down foodstuff is then swallowed, when it enters the stomach via the oesophagus. The mouth is surrounded by and contains the lips, gums, teeth, cheeks, tongue and palate. The space between the tongue and the palate is the cavity of the mouth and the space between the lips, gums and teeth and the cheeks is called the vestibule.

Lips

The lips form the orifice of the mouth. They form fleshy folds, which contain skeletal muscles and sensory receptors (Shier et al. 2004). These structures help in the assessment of the temperature and texture of foods eaten. The reddish colour of the lips results from numerous blood vessels. The junction between the upper and the lower lips forms the angle of the mouth.

Cheeks

These form the fleshy sides of the face and they run from the corner of the mouth to the side of the nose. Subcutaneous fat, muscles and mucous membranes line the cheeks. The cheeks assist in chewing food.

Palate

The palate is divided into two: the hard and the soft palate; both form the roof of the mouth whereas the tongue lies at the bottom of the oral cavity and forms the floor of the mouth. Both the hard palate and the soft palate are covered by mucous membranes.

Tongue

The tongue is a thick muscular organ composed of skeletal muscles and mucous membranes. It contains approximately 10 000 taste buds (Silverthorn 1998), which tell us about the taste of the food we eat, e.g. whether the food is sweet or sour. The tongue detects four basic tastes: sweet, salt, bitter and sour (Marieb 2004). Silverthorn (1998) identified a fifth taste called umami. This word is derived from the Japanese word meaning 'deliciousness', and the taste is associated with glutamate and some nucleotides. Hence, in some Asian countries monosodium glutamate (MSG) is sometimes used to enhance flavour when cooking (Silverthorn 1998).

The tongue is an accessory organ, which forms the floor of the mouth; it helps to blend food when chewing and to push food particles to the back of the mouth when swallowing. Tongue movement can alter the volume of the oral cavity and also has an important role in speech.

Teeth

Humans develop two sets of teeth: milk teeth and permanent teeth. There are about 20 milk teeth which begin to develop, usually, from the age of 6 months. Often one pair of milk teeth grows per month and they usually fall out between the ages of 6 and 12 years. Once the milk teeth fall out they are replaced by permanent teeth. Usually, there are 32 permanent teeth which have the potential to last a lifetime. However, permanent molars do not replace milk teeth. The first permanent molars appear at the age of 6 years, the second at the age of 12 years and the third may develop after the age of 13 years.

Figure 8.2
The regions of the stomach including the oesophagus and duodenum.

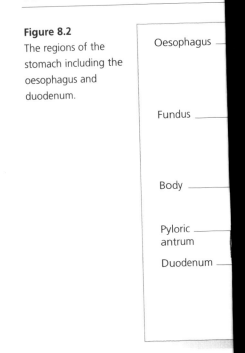

Oesophagus

Fundus

Body

Pyloric antrum

Duodenum

muscle layers in the stomach: longit
movement of the stomach is the ph

While in the stomach, various d
the food, thus helping chemical di
solid food particles are rendered i
pepsin will act on proteins and co
start the digestion of fats and renni
an insoluble form.

Summary of the functions of th

- Reservoir for food
- All food is liquefied, broken dov
- Proteins are converted into pep
- Milk is curdled and casein set fr
- Digestion of fats begins in the st
- Chyme is passed into the duode
- An anti-anaemic factor called vit

Small intestine

This is so named because of its d
intestine. It extends from the pylo
large intestine and is about 6 m in l

The small intestine is divided into three sections: the duodenum, jejunum and ileum. The duodenum is approximately 20 cm long and 5 cm in diameter (Shier et al. 2004), and is horseshoe shaped. The bile and pancreatic ducts open into the duodenum, approximately 10 cm from the pylorus, via the ampulla of Vater. It is through this channel that bile from the liver and the pancreatic juices enter the duodenum.

The jejunum is almost 2.5 m long and extends from the duodenum to the ileum (Marieb 2004). It occupies two-fifths of the small intestine and the ileum occupies the remaining three-fifths. There is no distinct separation between the jejunum and the ileum. However, the diameter of the jejunum is greater, and the wall of the jejunum is thicker, more vascular and more active compared with that of the ileum.

Large intestine

The large intestine is also known as the colon. It frames the small intestine and extends from the ileocaecal valve to the anus. Its diameter is greater than the small intestine but it is shorter in length: 1.5 m (Marieb 2004). The large intestine consists of the caecum, colon, rectum and anal canal. The colon is divided into the ascending, transverse, descending and sigmoid colons.

Summary of the functions of the colon

* Absorption of water and electrolytes
* Secretion of mucin
* Preparation of cellulose
* Defecation.

Other accessory organs

Salivary glands

These glands secrete saliva, which helps moisten food particles, binds them together and starts chemical digestion of carbohydrates. Saliva is watery and helps to maintain the pH in the mouth, which is alkaline, and to keep the mouth clean.

Liver

The liver is the largest gland in the body. It is situated in the upper right quadrant of the abdominal cavity beneath the diaphragm. It is partially protected by the ribs. The liver is reddish brown in colour and is a vascular organ. In an adult it weighs about 1.5 kg.

Some functions of the liver

* Aids metabolism of the body through chemical reactions from the absorbed nutrients

- Modifies waste products and toxic substances, i.e. drugs such as paracetamol, aspirin and alcohol
- Produces and stores glycogen
- Maintains blood sugar levels
- Produces bile, which emulsifies fats in the diet for absorption
- Forms urea, which is a waste product
- Forms red blood cells in fetal life
- Plays a part in the destruction of red blood cells
- Stores iron and the vitamins A, D and B_{12}
- Manufactures plasma proteins
- Produces prothrombins
- Produces anticoagulants.

Gallbladder

The gallbladder is a pear-shaped muscular sac, which lies beneath the liver. It is divided into the fundus, the body and the neck. The gallbladder is around 7-9 cm in length and its main function is to store and concentrate bile. The function of bile is to emulsify fats.

Pancreas

The pancreas is a triangular organ. It is more or less 12-15 cm in length and about 2.5 cm thick. It is divided into three parts: the head, body and tail. The head of the pancreas lies in the loop of the duodenum and the tail touches the spleen (Marieb 2004). It has two functions: exocrine and endocrine.

Exocrine functions

- Production of pancreatic juices
- Production of digestive enzymes, i.e. pancreatic amylase for the digestion of starch, trypsin for the digestion of proteins and lipase for the digestion of fats.

Endocrine functions

- Production of the hormone glucagon by the α cells
- Production of the hormone insulin by the β cells
- Production of the hormone somatostatin by the δ cells.

Care of patients with gastrointestinal disorders

Gingivitis

Also known as inflammation of the gums, gingivitis may lead to ulceration and necrosis of the gums. It may be caused by plaque, which is a sticky substance deposited on the exposed portions of the teeth, consisting of bacteria, food particles and mucus. Other possible causes of gingivitis are vigorous brushing and flossing of the teeth. Some individuals who have diabetes mellitus and certain pregnant women can develop gingivitis, which may be the result of hormonal changes (Kozier et al. 2004).

Predisposing factors

These may be caused by poor oral hygiene whereby bacteria infect the gums and the toxins produced by the bacteria cause the gingivitis. Long-term plaque deposits may also cause inflammation of the gums. Dental plaques are made up of mucin and colloid materials found in the saliva. They can mineralize into hard deposits called tartar and accumulate at the base of the teeth. Thus poor dental hygiene is also one of the causes of gingivitis. Certain drugs, e.g. phenytoin, some birth control pills and ingestion of heavy metals such as lead and bismuth may cause inflammation of the gums. Badly fitting orthodontic appliances, i.e. dentures, bridges and crowns, can irritate the gums and cause inflammation, leading to gingivitis.

Clinical symptoms

- Swollen and painful gums, tender when touched
- Bleeding from the gums and blood may be visible on the toothbrush even with gentle brushing
- Excessive salivation
- Bad breath (halitosis)
- Gums may appear shiny and/or bright red.

Treatment

A dentist should always be consulted when signs of gingivitis are suspected. The dentist may use dental instruments to remove the plaques and clean the teeth. Meticulous oral hygiene is essential after visiting the dentist. The dentist or the dental hygienist will demonstrate the correct method of brushing and flossing the teeth. The mouth should be rinsed using copious amounts of water after brushing and flossing.

The nurse should encourage those people who are at risk of contracting gingivitis to brush and floss their teeth after each meal. This will help to remove any food particles that may become lodged between the teeth.

Sialolithiasis

Sialolithiasis is the condition of stones in the salivary gland; it is the most common disease of the salivary gland (Iro et al. 1992). According to Cawson and Odell (1998), men are likely to be more affected than women, and children are rarely affected. Sialolithiasis generally occurs within the submaxillary gland. The stones are often made up of calcium oxalate and irregular in shape, although those in the ducts are small and oval in shape.

Predisposing factors

The exact aetiology and pathogenesis of sialolithiasis are unknown. However, sialolithiasis is thought to arise when the salivary glands are stagnated in calcium-rich saliva (Siddiqui 2002), which may be caused by:

• glandular infection
• inflammation of the ducts
• trauma to the ducts.

Clinical signs and symptoms

This condition is asymptomatic unless there is evidence of infection. The glands may be swollen and tender to the touch. Pain may occur at mealtimes when the salivary glands secrete saliva to lubricate the food for mastication and swallowing, and in response to other salivary stimuli. Other symptoms include palpable stones in the submandibular glands and excess salivation; some stones are visible on radiographs (Siddiqui 2002).

Treatment

Patients presenting with sialolithiasis may benefit from conservative treatment, especially when the stones are small. If the condition was caused by bacterial infection, a suitable antibiotic such as penicillin may be necessary as prescribed.

If the stones are large, they need to be removed surgically and in some cases, when the condition recurs, the affected gland may need to be removed. As Siddiqui (2002) suggests, the pain and swelling may be treated conservatively with medications such as non-steroidal anti-inflammatory drugs, e.g. ibuprofen.

Constipation

Constipation is the passing of hard and dry stools in small quantities. The frequency of the motion can be less than three times a week (Lemone and Burke 2004). The causes of constipation are many and varied and may result from life-style or organic diseases or be related to functional disorders of the colon.

Predisposing factors

Poor dietary habits can lead to constipation when the diet is highly refined, with very little fibre and inadequate fluid intake. Fibre in the diet helps to form faecal bulk and water helps to keep the stool soft. Diseases of the large bowel, e.g. tumours, adhesions, diverticular disease and anal strictures, are some of the pathological problems that could cause constipation. Opioid drugs, e.g. morphine, may cause constipation (Lemone and Burke 2004). Patients should be advised of the potential side effects and what they might do to avoid constipation. Other factors associated with constipation include:

- poor fluid intake
- lack of exercise
- neurological disorders such as multiple sclerosis
- psychological problems, e.g. depression
- clinical signs and symptoms
- abdominal pain
- abdominal distension
- loss of appetite
- nausea and vomiting in some patients
- hard and dry faecal matter (if produced).

Nursing management

The patient must be assessed carefully by the nurse to ascertain his or her food likes and dislikes, and to attempt to identify the cause of the constipation. If the cause is a dietary problem, food high in fibre should be recommended. Vegetables and fresh fruits are a good source of fibre and should form part of the diet (Winney 1998). Fibre helps to form bulk and draws water into the stool, which helps to soften the stool and make defecation easier.

Peate (2003) states that bulk laxatives such as Fybogel are the first line of treatment when managing constipation. They help peristalsis of the colon and thus reduce the time the faeces take to move through the colon. However, McCuistion and Gutierrez (2002) state that bulk laxatives should not be given to patients with gastrointestinal disorders such as bowel obstruction or acute abdominal pain or those who have had recent bowel surgery.

If necessary, laxatives, e.g. lactulose, suppositories or phosphate enemas, may be given to assist in bowel evacuation; these medications need to be prescribed by the doctor, before administration. The patient should be encouraged by the nurse to drink at least 2000–3000 ml fluid daily for normal faecal elimination (Kozier et al. 2004). This daily intake of fluid would increase the water content of chyme, which may move chyme more quickly in the large intestine; this gives less time for fluid absorption to take place and as a result the stool will be soft (Kozier et al. 2004).

Mobilization such as walking should be encouraged if this is not contraindicated; if this is not permissible, chair-bound exercises such as stretching will help to strengthen abdominal muscles and aid peristalsis of the colon, which facilitates elimination of stool (Winney 1998).

Enemas

An enema is the insertion of liquid into the colon or rectum. There are various types of enemas available, including cleansing and retention enemas (Smith et al. 2004). Enemas must be prescribed before administration.

Reasons for administering enemas

There are several reasons for the administration of an enema, e.g. to encourage bowel movements in patients who are constipated. Enemas are also given to patients before bowel surgery such as the formation of a colostomy, and before certain investigations, e.g. sigmoidoscopy.

Nursing management

The nurse must always explain the procedure to the patient in order to ascertain that he or she understands what is to be done and the reason why it is necessary to administer the enema. The bed should be screened in order to ensure privacy. If possible ask the patient to empty the bladder because this may reduce discomfort during the procedure. Read the label fully and follow the manufacturer's instructions. Warm the fluid to body temperature of between 36.5 and 37°C in a bowl of warm water. Lie the patient on the left side in the Sims' position – this is a position in which the patient lies on the left side with the right knee and thigh drawn upward towards the chest. This facilitates easy insertion of fluid into the rectum and the flow of fluid by gravity into the sigmoid and descending colon (Kozier et al. 2004). Place a protective sheet under the patient's buttocks to protect the bed linen from any spillages.

Wash hands, don gloves and observe infection control procedures as suggested in the local procedure and policy. Lubricate the tip of the enema with lubricant and squeeze the enema to expel the air in the bag. Introducing air into the rectum during the procedure may cause discomfort to the patient.

Gently insert the enema into the rectum and squeeze the bag to insert the fluid. Observe the patient for discomfort and pain at all times during the procedure. On completion, gently remove the enema from the rectum while at the same time keeping the bag squeezed or rolled up when removing from the rectum. This prevents the liquid from flowing back into the bag. Wipe the patient's anal area with tissue and encourage the patient to retain the enema for the appropriate amount of time, e.g. 5-10 minutes for cleansing enemas and 30 minutes for retention enemas (Kozier et al. 2004).

Ensure that the patient is comfortable, dispose of equipment safely and wash your hands. When the patient is ready to defecate, assist the patient to the toilet, if possible, or give a bedpan or a bedside commode. Document the outcome of the procedure in the nursing care plan. Nurses need to be aware that in undertaking this procedure they are accountable for their actions and that documentation is in accord with the *Code of Professional Conduct* (NMC 2002).

Suppositories

Reasons for inserting suppositories

Administration of medications into the rectum is a common practice (Kozier et al. 2004). Suppositories are given to patients who are constipated to induce bowel movement, to evacuate the bowel before surgery and to administer medications such as antibiotics or analgesics (Jamieson et al. 2002) and for patients who are vomiting and therefore cannot take oral medications or those who may have difficulty swallowing.

Nursing management

Explain the procedure to the patient to gain consent and cooperation for inserting the suppository. The bed should be screened in order to provide privacy; this may also encourage the patient to relax. Place a protective sheet under the patient's buttocks, in case of soiling by stool at the time of insertion of the suppository (Jamieson et al. 2002). Put a glove on the hand used to insert the suppository. Check the prescription chart to ensure that the suppository has been prescribed, the correct patient is receiving the suppository and the dose is what has been prescribed.

Ask the patient to lie on the left side and gently insert the suppository about 6 cm into the rectum. Moppett (2000) suggests that the blunt end of the suppository should be inserted first because this will help with retention of the suppository as the muscles of the anal sphincter close tightly around the pointed end, thus helping it to move up into the rectum.

Remove your finger after insertion and wipe the patient's anal region with a tissue. Ask the patient to retain the suppository for at least 30 minutes, or according to the manufacturer's recommendations, before he or she evacuates the contents of the rectum. Dispose of used equipment safely and wash your hands. When the need arises to evacuate, assist the patient to the toilet or offer a bedpan or commode, ensuring privacy at all times. Document the outcome in the nursing care plan.

Colostomy

Colostomy is a surgical procedure where an artificial opening (stoma) is created on the abdomen to allow the drainage of stool from the colon. It could be either temporary or permanent. The stoma serves an artificial anus through which the colon can empty the waste products of digestion. A stoma bag is applied to the colostomy where faecal matter can be collected (Smith et al. 2004) (Figure 8.3).

Reasons for colostomy formation

- When the colon, rectum or the anus do not function normally, e.g. in cancer of the large bowel, ulcerative colitis and Crohn's disease.
- When the colon, rectum or anus needs to rest for a period of time. This may be caused by inflammation or oedema of the large intestine.
- In certain conditions such as Hirschsprung's disease – a condition in which the nerves controlling bowel function are abnormal – or in imperforate anus – an absence of anal opening.
- In severe abdominal injuries, e.g. after road traffic accident and in patients who have had radiation therapy.

Figure 8.3
Three different sites of stoma: end-ileostomy, transverse loop colostomy and end colostomy.

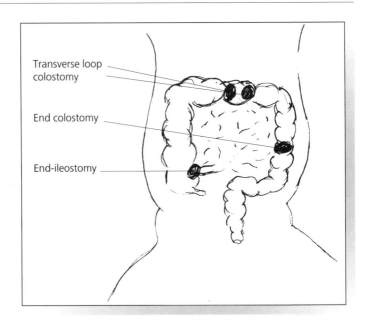

Transverse loop colostomy

End colostomy

End-ileostomy

Sites to be avoided when siting stoma

- Umbilical region
- Hip bones
- Old scar/surgical incisions
- Waist line
- Pubic area
- Uneven skin folds
- Groin crease.

Nursing management

A full preoperative assessment is essential to ensure that the patient clearly understands the nature of the surgery and for any questions that the patient may want answered. Helping patients to adjust to altered body image can lead to uneventful recovery postoperatively (Allison and Stuchfield 1994).

Postoperatively, it is also essential to observe the stoma site for bleeding, infection or any other problems such as retraction of the stoma. It is common to find some blood in the ostomy bag in the early postoperative days (Lemone and Burke 2004). The stoma should appear pink and moist. The nurse must maintain skin integrity by ensuring that the stoma appliance fits well on to the stoma without any leakage, ensuring that the skin surrounding the stoma site is clean and dry, and providing skin barrier cream if necessary.

The contents of the bag should be observed and any changes such as retraction of the stoma reported to the nurse in charge. Patient education in the care of stoma, such as the emptying of the bag when necessary, applying the pouch clamp and changing the stoma bag, aids acceptance of the stoma and promotion of independence in the patient (Finlay 2002). Whether the stoma is temporary or permanent, ultimately the patient will be responsible for stoma management when discharged.

Changes in dietary habit are not necessary after the formation of a colostomy. If the patient is concerned about an offensive stool and the build-up of gases in the bag some dietary advice from the dietitian may help (Marjoram 1999).

Any changes must be documented accordingly and nursing care plans should be updated as necessary; it is the nurse's responsibility to ensure that all records are accurate and up to date (NMC 2002).

Discharge planning

- Discuss with both patient and relatives (if appropriate) how to cope with a colostomy
- Arrange home visits by the stoma care nurse
- Provide details about relevant agencies/voluntary agencies
- Dietary advice if necessary
- Letter for general practitioner and district nurse
- Out-patient appointment
- Medications to take home if necessary
- Ensure a good supply of stoma appliances.

Renal system

The renal system consists of the kidneys, ureters, bladder and urethra. These structures ensure that a stable internal environment is maintained for the survival of cells and tissues in the body – homeostasis.

There are two kidneys, one on each side of the spinal column. They are approximately 11 cm long, 5–6 cm wide and 3–4 cm thick (Marieb 2004). They are said to be 'bean-shaped' organs where the outer border is convex; the inner border is known as the hilum, and it is here that the renal arteries enter the kidneys. The functional units of the kidneys are called the nephrons and there are about 1.2 million nephrons in each kidney. The kidneys produce urine by filtering blood, which is then channelled into the bladder by the ureters (Marieb 2004) (Figure 8.4).

The bladder, a pear-shaped organ, lies in the pelvic cavity. It contains smooth muscle fibres, which stretch as the bladder fills with urine. The position of the bladder varies with age. In infants and younger children the bladder is slightly raised, whereas in adults it lies in the pelvis. It lies in front of the rectum and in women it lies in front of the uterus. The bladder has a good supply of blood vessels so it bleeds heavily in trauma and bladder surgery. Urine is conveyed from the bladder to the exterior by the urethra.

Figure 8.4 Aspects of
the renal system and
associated structures.

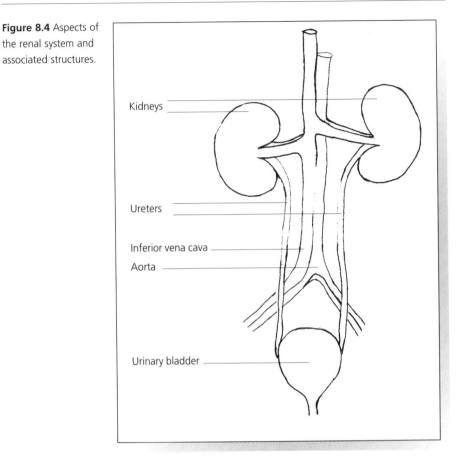

Kidneys

Ureters

Inferior vena cava

Aorta

Urinary bladder

Functions of the kidneys

- Excrete urine and waste products such as urea, uric acid and creatinine
- Regulate fluid balance
- Regulate electrolyte balance
- Maintain pH of the blood
- Secrete rennin, which helps to regulate blood pressure
- Secrete erythropoietin, which stimulates the production of red blood cells.

The prostate gland

Although the prostate gland is not part of the renal system, it does play a part in issues related to elimination of the bladder, hence the reason for discussion of the prostate gland in this section. The prostate is the size of a walnut. It lies below the bladder, surrounding the urethra. The gland is very vascular and plays a major role in the male reproductive system. It secretes a thin, milky, alkaline substance which contains two enzymes, namely fibrinolysin and acid phosphatase (Clancy and McVicar 1995). These enzymes help in the motility of the sperm. Enlargement of this gland, whether malignant or benign, can cause retention of urine.

Care of patients with urological disorders

Retention of urine

Retention of urine is the inability to pass urine despite the desire to urinate. If untreated, in the long term urinary retention can cause bladder enlargement and severe cases can affect the ureters and the kidneys, namely hydroureter and hydronephrosis (Lemone and Burke 2004). There are many reasons why individuals cannot void urine.

Causes of retention of urine

- Enlarged prostate gland causing stricture of the urethra
- Urethral stricture resulting from trauma, urinary tract infection and bladder calculi
- Certain drugs, e.g. antihistamines, antidepressants or antipsychotics
- Some surgery adjacent to the urethra, e.g. abdominoperineal resection
- Neurogenic bladder, caused by disruption of the nerves to the bladder, multiple sclerosis or faecal impaction, can lead to the retention of urine.

Signs and symptoms

Patients may complain of nocturia, i.e. getting up two or more times during the night to pass urine. They may have difficulty in passing urine (dysuria) and may find that they cannot empty their bladder fully (Kumar and Clark 2002). The patient may complain of 'dribbling', leading to urine-stained clothing. Incomplete emptying of the bladder can lead to over-distension causing loss of muscle tone to the bladder. Haematuria may be present in the urine as a result of stricture of the urethra (Fickenscher 1999).

Nursing management

The nurse must undertake a full assessment of the patient and establish when he or she last passed urine. The nurse should obtain a full nursing history in order to establish the cause of retention before treating the patient. If urinary retention was not the result of mechanical obstructions such as an enlarged prostate or stricture of the urethra, the nurse may attempt to relax the patient. If necessary the nurse may need to assist the patient to the toilet so that he or she can have some privacy when attempting to void urine. For some patients the sound of running water from a tap may encourage them to pass urine.

Some patients may find it difficult to pass urine postoperatively, which may be the result of pain from the surgical incision, or they may find it difficult to pass urine when they are lying down in bed. The nurse should determine whether the patient is in any pain and if so provide the prescribed analgesia in order to attempt to relax the patient.

If the above measures fail, then the patient may need to be catheterized in order to empty his or her bladder artificially. The nurse should observe strict aseptic technique when catheterizing a patient and must adhere to local policy and procedures related to the catheterization of a patient. When the catheter is *in situ* encourage the patient to drink at least 2.5 l of fluid per day, providing that the patient is not suffering from other physiological problems such as congestive cardiac failure (Wilson 2001).

An accurate record of all fluid intake and urine output must be maintained and recorded on a fluid balance chart; all nurses caring for the patient should be made aware of the importance of maintaining an accurate fluid balance chart (Walsh 2002).

Discharge planning

The patient may be discharged once the cause of the retention of urine is resolved and the patient is able to void urine without the assistance of a urinary catheter. The patient should be encouraged to maintain his or her fluid intake of at least 2.5 l per day. This would promote constant urinary production, which may help to prevent urinary tract infection (Wilson 2001). Encourage the patient to visit the toilet regularly to void and not to ignore the urge to micturate. This could prevent urinary tract infection and the development of an atonic bladder, which could in turn lead to retention of urine.

Bladder irrigation

Bladder irrigation is performed using a three-way urinary catheter. This procedure is undertaken in patients who have undergone, for example, transurethral resection of the prostate gland (TURP). The prostate gland becomes enlarged as a result of a malignancy or for benign reasons. Patients with an enlarged prostate gland may experience difficulty in voiding urine and can develop urine retention. These patients may need to undergo TURP to alleviate the problem. After a TURP patients usually return to the ward with bladder irrigation *in situ*; bladder irrigation is used postoperatively primarily to remove debris from the bladder (Walsh 2002).

Nursing management

Check to ensure that the irrigating fluid is running as prescribed. The drip rate of the irrigating fluid can be adjusted by the roller clamp on the tubing of the giving set. The rate should be adjusted according to the colour of the urine in the catheter bag (Smith et al. 2004). The nurse should increase the rate of fluid if the urinary output is dark red and contains blood clots, and decrease the flow rate if the output is pink and clear of clots. The irrigation system must be a closed continuous system and the nurse must ensure that there is no leaking at the connections. The patient is assessed by the nurse, every hour, to ensure that he is not in any discomfort as a result of retention of urine or pain related to surgery.

The drainage systems should be checked half hourly for the first 36–48 hours for patency (Walsh 2002). The colour, consistency or sediment in the drainage should be noted. The urine will be blood stained for at least the first 24 hours and will gradually become less blood stained. The nurse must empty the catheter bag when needed and maintain a fluid balance chart. It is important to observe that the volume drained is the same as the volume used for irrigation, plus any urine that may be produced. If the volume drained is less than the volume instilled, the nurse in charge must be informed immediately. The rationale for the reduced drainage may be the result of obstruction of the drainage tube by a blood clot, which could lead to retention of urine and discomfort for the patient.

Once the patient is fully conscious and able to tolerate fluids, unless contraindicated the nurse should encourage the patient to drink and gradually increase fluid intake to at least 2–2.5 l fluid/day. Once the patient is tolerating fluids, bladder irrigation should be discontinued if the urine output is free of blood clots and the urine draining freely into the urinary drainage bag. Catheter care, as described below, should be provided daily to help to prevent infection.

Discharge planning

• Encourage the patient to continue taking 2.5 l fluid daily to ensure that the urine output is clear.
• Ask the patient to observe the colour of the urine. If bleeding is observed, he or she should consult a doctor immediately.
• Avoid becoming constipated because straining during defecation could put pressure on the urethral passage and cause bleeding (Walsh 2002).
• Some would suggest that patients should avoid sex for about 3 weeks.

Catheter care

Urinary catheters are used to remove urine from the bladder or instil fluid or drugs into the bladder. Urinary catheters come in various sizes and there are different types of catheter made from different types of materials. When catheterizing a patient, nurses should ensure that they use the correct size catheter, e.g. 12–14 Fr (Ch) (Marjoram 1999). An incorrect catheter size may result in damage to the urethra during insertion and can cause urethral scarring and stricture.

Reasons for catheterization

- Acute or chronic urinary retention
- Preoperatively and postoperatively in abdominal, rectal and pelvic surgeries
- For administration of drug treatments, e.g. cytotoxic drugs
- To irrigate the bladder to remove blood clots or sediment.

Table 8.1 lists the various types of catheter. Teflon-coated catheters reduce urethral irritation and may be used for patients who need short- to medium-term catheterization; this type of catheter may remain *in situ* for up to 1 month. Silicone catheters have a longer lifespan compared with Teflon-coated catheters; they may remain *in situ* for about 3 months. The hydrogel catheters absorb water and cause less friction when catheterizing a patient. These catheters may last *in situ* for up to 4 months (Marjoram 1999) (Figure 8.5).

Table 8.1 Various types of catheters

Type	Description
Teflon	The rubber is Teflon coated Short to medium term
Silicone	Soft and causes less irritation Catheter may be left *in situ* for up to 3 months
Hydrogel	Absorbs water and is easy to insert Lasts up to 14 weeks

Nursing management

Patients with a urinary catheter *in situ* should be encouraged to drink at least 2.5 l fluid/day, providing they do not have other physiological problems such as cardiac failure. About 2–2.5 l fluid normally results in an increase in urine production, which in turn will help to prevent urinary tract infection; it is important that the nurse maintains a strict fluid balance chart – monitoring input and output.

   If necessary, daily meatal hygiene should be undertaken to ensure that the patient does not develop a urinary tract infection. For uncircumcised males, gently retract the foreskin over the head of the penis away from the catheter. Using soap and clean water cleanse around the meatus. Gently apply torsion to the catheter and clean away from the tip of the penis where the catheter enters it, wiping 7–10 cm down the tubing towards the catheter bag (Smith et al. 2004).

   Strict asepsis should be observed when cleaning the meatus of the penis, so as not to introduce any infection into the bladder. Ensure that the catheter bag is not lying on the floor and that it is attached to a catheter bag stand;

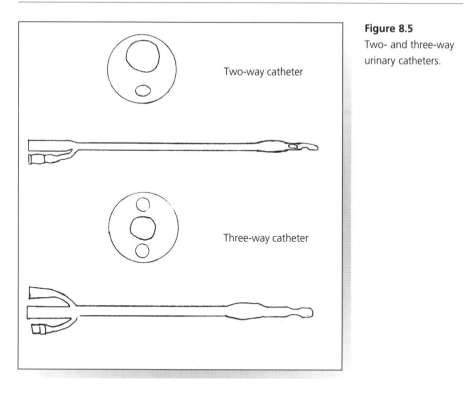

Figure 8.5
Two- and three-way
urinary catheters.

furthermore, make certain that there are no kinks in the catheter drainage
system which might prevent the urine from flowing unimpeded into the bag
(Smith et al. 2004).

All care and outcomes must be documented accordingly, to ensure that
the care provided is based on an individual assessment of the patient's needs.

Conclusions

The overall aim of this chapter was to provide the reader with insight into
some of the problems associated with elimination and the care of a patient
with certain disorders associated with the alimentary and eliminatory
tracts. The content of this chapter includes disorders of the gastrointestinal
tract and the urinary system. It is not possible to include all the disorders
related to these areas, but some of the more common problems have been
discussed.

Attending to the patient's elimination needs is an important part of
holistic care. Nurses are often involved in assisting or giving advice to
patients who have elimination problems. These problems could affect the
patient both psychologically and physically. The inability to defecate and
urinate may be caused by various disorders, e.g. carcinoma. These disorders
may impinge on the patient's ability to perform activities of living.

Some patients may need assistance with defecation in the form of suppositories or an enema, whereas others may need a colostomy as a result of cancer of the colon. Patients who are catheterized for urinary problems such as retention of urine, or male patients who have had a prostatectomy and have a catheter *in situ*, will need catheter care in order to prevent urinary tract infection. The nurse must provide evidence-based care. Care must be provided as a result of individual, holistic assessment.

References

Allison, M. and Stuchfield, B. (1994) Helping to adjust: an holistic approach to stoma care. RCN nursing update supplement. Nursing Standard 8(36): 3–8.

Cawson, R.A. and Odell, E.W. (1998) Essentials of Oral Pathology and Oral Medicine, 6th edn. Edinburgh: Churchill Livingstone.

Clancy, J. and McVicar, A.J. (1995) Physiology and Anatomy: A homeostatic approach. London: Edward Arnold.

Fickenscher, L. (1999) Evaluation of adult haematuria. Nurse Practitioner 24(9): 58–64.

Finlay, T. (2002) Caring for the patient with a disorder of the gastrointestinal system. In: Walsh, M. (ed.), Watson's Clinical Nursing and Related Sciences, 6th edn. London: Baillière Tindall, pp. 435–506.

Iro, H., Schneider, H.Th., Fodra, C. et al. (1992) Shockwave lithotripsy of salivary duct stones. Lancet 339: 1333–1336.

Jamieson, E.M., McCall, J.M. and Whyte, L.A. (2002) Clinical Nursing Practice, 4th edn. Edinburgh: Churchill Livingstone.

Kozier, B., Erb, G., Berman, A. and Synder, S.J. (2004) Fundamentals of Nursing, 7th edn. Englewood Cliffs, NJ: Pearson Prentice Hall.

Kumar, P. and Clark, M. (2002) Clinical Medicine, 5th edn. London: W.B. Saunders.

Lemone, P. and Burke, K. (2004) Medical–Surgical Nursing: Critical thinking in client care, 3rd edn. Englewood Cliffs, NJ: Pearson Prentice Hall.

McCuistion, L.E. and Gutierrez, K.J. (2002) Pharmacology. Philadelphia: WB Saunders.

Mader, S.S. (1997) Understanding Human Anatomy and Physiology, 3rd edn. London: Wm C. Brown Publishers.

Marieb, E.N. (2004) Human Anatomy and Physiology, 6th edn. San Francisco, CA: Pearson Benjamin Cummings.

Marjoram, B. (1999) Elimination. In: Hogston, R. and Simpson, P.M. (eds), Foundations of Nursing Practice. London: Macmillan, pp. 149–184.

Moppett, S. (2000) Which way is up for a suppository? Nursing Times Plus 96(19): 12–13.

Nursing and Midwifery Council (2002) Code of Professional Conduct. London: NMC.

Peate, I. (2003) Nursing role in the management of constipation: use of laxatives. British Journal of Nursing 12: 1130–1136.

Shier, D., Butler, J. and Lewis, R. (2004) Holes Human Anatomy and Physiology, 10th edn. London: McGraw Hill.

Siddiqui, S.J. (2002) Sialolithiasis: an unusually large submandibular salivary stone. British Dental Journal 193: 89–91.

Silverthorn, D.U. (1998) Human Physiology: An integrated approach. Englewood Cliffs, NJ: Prentice Hall.

Smith, S.F., Duell, D.J. and Martin, B.C. (2004) Clinical Nursing Skills: Basic to advanced skills, 6th edn. Englewood Cliffs, NJ: Pearson Prentice Hall.

Walsh, M. (2002) Watson's Clinical Nursing and Related Sciences, 6th edn. London: Baillière Tindall.

Wilson, J. (2001) Infection Control in Clinical Practice, 2nd edn. London: Baillière Tindall.

Winney, J. (1998) Constipation. Nursing Standard 13(11): 49–53.

CHAPTER 9

Personal cleansing and dressing

LAUREEN HEMMING

Caring for personal hygiene is often an activity carried out in private and determined by personal preference; usually, the products used are a matter of individual choice and may be determined by what is affordable and available. Some people prefer showering to bathing; how often and when are matters of personal choice, which may be determined by the weather - in hot seasons or countries, people may wash or shower more frequently. However, this may be determined by the availability of water: in drought, people are urged to minimize its use (Roper et al. 1996). For some, however, these practices, such as washing in running water, and the products used may be determined culturally or by personal beliefs, e.g. some vegetarians or vegans will not use soaps made from animal products containing tallow. The Nursing and Midwifery Council (NMC 2002) stipulates that all nurses, midwives and health visitors must respect a patient's personal choice.

The skin is the largest organ of the body (Lewis and Roberts 1998, Martini et al. 1998); it forms a protective barrier and can be harmed through neglect or exposure to the elements. There are many factors affecting skin condition: state of health, age, diet, the pollutants in the atmosphere, the irritants that may be applied to the skin in the process of personal cleansing, the weather - sun, wind, snow and ice. People in the northern hemisphere are more likely to experience dry skin in winter, especially when climatic temperatures fall below skin temperature. Ersser and Penzer (2000) point out that skin diseases are a problem all over the world, although their causes and outcomes may be very different in different countries; it is an area in which nurses are best placed to help in providing direct care, health education and support. They report that 70% of the population in developing countries suffer from skin disease and many cannot access the requirements for basic skin care.

The most common diseases are infestation and opportunist bacterial infections (Table 9.1). Ersser and Penzer (2000) write:

> The promotion of healthy skin is a fundamental concern of nursing in almost all speciality areas. By maintaining healthy skin to serve as a disease barrier, nurses

Table 9.1 Skin diseases in different parts of the world

Skin diseases of developed countries	Skin diseases of developing countries
Chronic skin conditions	Infections
Inflammatory diseases	Infestations
Eczema	Scabies
Psoriasis	Fungal infections
	Bacterial infections

From Ersser and Penzer (2000).

not only help to manage acute and chronic skin disease but also help to prevent and manage pressure sores and wounds.

They believe that a great deal of suffering can be managed by appropriate nursing care because they require low-technology health-care strategies to combat problems. Nurses can advise on skin hygiene, the use of moisturizers and measures to protect against sunburn, and give dietary advice.

Disease and illness can cause the patient to feel unclean and dirty; the desire to be cleansed extends beyond the mere washing of the skin. Patients with a diagnosis of cancer may claim to feel contaminated and dirty; similarly, people who have been abused instinctively want to wash before they report the abuse perpetrated against them. Thus the ritual of washing takes on symbolic significance. Although washing the patient does not eliminate the disease or abuse, it does make her or him feel better. The act of assisting in personal cleansing works not only on the physical level but also on the psychological and spiritual levels (Collins and Hampton 2003).

What we wear, the clothes we put on, after the routine of personal cleansing is also a matter of personal choice; however, this choice may be influenced by cultural expectations and beliefs about decency and what is appropriate for a person to wear in a given community. The clothing that we select may give an indication of our social status, our level of income; it may denote aspects of our personality and extraverts may dress more flamboyantly than introverts. For some teenagers, it may not be about what is worn, but about whether it has been manufactured by the 'cool' company, whether the right logo is attached. The clothing chosen by teenagers often provides them with a group identity and a social structure. The wearing of a uniform may denote where we work and in what capacity. It is not just the employees in public services who have to wear a uniform. Some large retail outlets expect employees to wear a uniform correctly because it gives them a sense of corporate identity and makes a statement to the public about the environment, value and safety of the products that they are selling, or the service they are providing. Sometimes uniform is worn to protect the wearer and sometimes it is worn to protect the public who come into contact with the wearer. Plastic aprons and gloves are used for protection and to minimize the risks of cross-infection (Peto 1998).

This chapter is concerned with a brief anatomy and physiology of the skin, some of the common issues associated with maintaining a healthy skin, and the nursing care required particularly when an individual cannot meet his or her own hygiene needs.

Anatomy and physiology of the skin

The skin or integumentary system is the largest organ of the body and the only visible one, made up of the cutaneous membrane that is the skin and the accessory structures - the hair and nails (Martini et al. 1998). The skin has several functions:

- Protects the internal tissues and organs
- Excretes water - about 500 ml is lost a day through the skin, taking with it salts and organic waste products, and known as insensible loss
- Stores nutrients
- Necessary for the synthesis of vitamin D when exposed to sunlight
- Detects sensations such as touch, pain, pressure and temperature
- Maintains body temperature.

The skin consists of two layers: the dermis or inner layer and the epidermis or outer layer. Under these two layers is a third layer called the subcutaneous membrane, sometimes referred to as the hypodermis or the superficial fascia. Clancy and McVicar (1995) believe that, as the cells in the subcutaneous membrane do not generate the cells of the dermis and epidermis, this layer is separate from the other two; however, this layer acts as a protective barrier to the internal organs.

The epidermis

The epidermis mainly has four layers of cells; on the soles of the feet and the palms of the hands there is an additional layer of cells. The cell thickness of each layer varies, with more exposed skin being thicker than unexposed skin.

The basal layer of the epidermis, called the stratum germinativum or stratum basale, is the layer that produces the skin cells, which migrate outwards to form the outer layer of skin. These layers form genetically defined ridges, which are unique to each person, and are visible at the fingertips - hence the use of fingerprints to help solve crimes. Within this layer, Merkel cells are found which are sensitive to touch and pressure. This layer becomes thinner as we age, which is why the skin in older people becomes more delicate and more easily damaged, and requires more care (Collins and Hampton 2003).

The next layer consists of eight to ten layers of cells called the stratum spinosum. The cells are characteristically prickly or spiny and are held together by desmosomes – a very strong intercellular cement-type protein. Within this layer are Langerhans' cells, which produce an immune response when the skin is damaged.

The stratum granulosum has a depth of three to five cells and produces keratin, which is needed for the production of hair and nails. In the soles of the feet and the palms of the hand only, the next layer is the stratum lucidum; this consists of clear hard cells that are filled with keratin to give extra protection.

The final layer is the stratum corneum, believed by Martini et al. (1998) to be 15–30 layers deep. It takes the cells about 15–30 days to reach the outer layers and cells remain on the outer layer for about 2 weeks. Brushing the skin with a soft bristle brush using short strokes will remove the most outer layer of cells. The brushing is invigorating and stimulates the underlying blood circulation, thus improving tone and colour. Clancy and McVicar (1995) and Martini et al. (1998) suggest that the cells in the stratum corneum are dead, but more recent research (Johnson 2004) suggests that these cells should not be viewed as such. Johnson (2004) claims that:

> the stratum corneum is not an inert protective barrier, but a most elegantly designed and dynamic structure.

The cells in the stratum corneum, as they reach the surface, become flatter and dryer; the dry surface prevents the growth of micro-organisms, however, and if this layer becomes too dry other skin problems occur. This protection from micro-organisms is aided by the production of sebum from sebaceous glands in the dermis that open out onto the epidermis, which gives the skin surface an oily covering. The stratum corneum is water resistant but not waterproof. When the skin is immersed in clean fresh water as in a bath, water enters the cells through the process of osmosis. The cells can absorb four times their normal volume.

After-wash skin tightness

Use of some kinds of soaps has the same effect on the skin as swimming in the sea, in that the lather produced by the soap while on the skin has a higher concentration and thus draws water out of the epidermis. This is referred to as transepidermal water loss (TEWL) (Lodén et al. 2003), or after-wash tightness (AWT) (Ananthapadmanabhan et al. 2004). The very product that is used to promote cleanliness and clean the skin can have damaging effects on the skin and lead to the development of conditions such as acute dermatitis and eczema. Soaps affect the stratum corneum's protein balance and damage to the proteins affects the body's own natural moisturizing factor. As the skin dries, the water loss from the stratum corneum is felt as tautness, and the skin looks shiny and tight. To combat this, manufacturers of soaps and other cleansing products are introducing moisturizers to soften and protect the skin. While the skin is taut, it is more easily damaged, so a supple skin is more resilient and less likely to be damaged (Collins and Hampton 2003, Rawlings 2003).

The dermis

The dermis has two layers: next to the epidermis is the papillary layer. It folds and follows the folds of the stratum germinativum, its blood capillaries providing the stratum germinativum with a blood supply. The layer is made up of loose connective tissue which contains sensory nerve fibres as well as the blood capillaries.

Under this lies the reticular layer, which is made up of collagen fibres, elastin and connective tissue. The collagen and elastin fibres give skin its durability and elasticity. The collagen fibres run through the dermis into the epidermis and, at the other end, into the subcutaneous tissue. The collagen fibres form rough bundles, which flow in a given direction, called lines of cleavage. If a surgeon cuts along the lines of cleavage, when the wound heals there is little scarring. Cutting across the lines of cleavage inevitably leads to more pronounced scarring. Collagen and elastin in the dermis alter with age and are damaged by hormones and ultraviolet radiation, leaving the skin wrinkled (Malik 1998, Rawlings 2003).

Within the dermis there are hair follicles, glands, blood vessels and nerve fibres. The nerve fibres are sensitive to pressure, pain and temperature, and they also adjust the secretions from the sweat glands. There are three types of glands in the skin: sebaceous, sweat and ceruminous glands. Sebaceous glands secrete sebum, an oily substance containing cholesterol, fatty acids, proteins, salts and bactericidal chemicals. These glands lie close to the hair follicles. Sweat glands are either apocrine or eccrine. The apocrine glands are mainly in the axilla and the pubic region, and their secretions contain pheromones - a scent that is sexually stimulating. The eccrine glands secrete a watery substance, which contains waste products. Ceruminous glands line the ear and produce wax, which has a protective function. If the secretions from the glands remain on the skin surface they attract bacteria and this changes their composition and can cause odour, hence the need for washing and maintaining personal hygiene (Collins and Hampton 2003).

Cultural perspectives

There are rituals involving cleansing that have a symbolic significance; the person is cleansed of their 'sin' through baptism, or they are cleansed as an act of purification. In some religions, the event, as in Christian baptism, may occur only once, but in other religions, such as Islam and Judaism, cleansing may form part of a daily ritual. Malik (1998) points out that the ancient civilizations of Greece, Rome and Egypt introduced hygiene and cleanliness, but these practices changed through the Middle Ages, particularly in Europe, where spiritual purity was considered more important than physical cleanliness; indeed washing could expose one to illness. Spiritual purity was achieved through other means such as being involved in good works. The use of hot water at this time was considered to open up the pores in the skin and leave one susceptible to infection. Over time, practices have changed; where once houses in the UK were built without bathrooms, now most have more than one room allocated to washing; the master bedroom may even have en suite facilities.

Islam is more than a religion, it is a way of life, and Islamic teaching includes guidance on social behaviours, observances and practices, which assist the individual in developing a healthy lifestyle. Besides declaring their faith, engaging in prayer, fasting and making a pilgrimage to Mecca, Muslims are expected to engage in self-purification. Self-purification involves more than just personal cleanliness; it requires the setting aside of a proportion of wealth for the needy. Fasting is also a means of self-purification and good for health (Rassool 2000).

Muslims are expected to maintain a high standard of personal hygiene not merely from a physical need but because this also has spiritual significance. The ritual of washing needs to be performed before any other act or behaviour, such as eating or praying. When Muslims are ill and confined to bed, they will require assistance to perform this throughout the day. Cleanliness extends beyond keeping the body clean, to keeping the internal aspect of the body clean – this means not eating food considered to be unclean, e.g. pork or pork products, meat of dead animals, their blood, or drinking alcohol. Rassool (2000) explains that washing has a symbolic significance. Illness is perceived as a means whereby the sufferer can be cleansed on a physical, emotional, spiritual and mental level; it is a way in which one can atone for one's sins. This does not mean that a Muslim will not seek remedial therapies; however, Muslims will abstain from medication that includes alcohol or pork products. The rituals around cleanliness are important and must be maintained. Thus, when Muslims are patients they require access to running water for washing, and need to be able to wash as and when necessary. However, although personal preferences are to be respected, the nurse should not assume that, as a patient is a Muslim, all of the above applies. Nor should the nurse assume that, if the patients are of Asian or Arabic origin, they are also Muslim. Gerrish (2000) points out that nurses frequently do not ask patients what their preferences may be:

> Ethnic categories, however carefully defined do not correspond with cultural, linguistic, dietary or religious preferences and needs.

Some cultures and social groups have strict guidelines on what clothing is worn. Malik (1998) and Rees (1997) both describe that total removal of all objects and items of clothing for cleansing purposes is not permitted in some religions. Most Sikhs wear five items that are symbols of their religion:

(1) the kais (uncut hair)
(2) a kanga (a comb)
(3) kaccha (underwear – loose pants)
(4) a kara (a bangle)
(5) a kirpan (a small dagger).

Even when changing from one pair of kaccha to a clean pair, the soiled ones are not removed totally; one leg remains inside one pair while the other leg is placed in the clean pair, and as the soiled pants are removed then the second leg is inserted.

Martini et al. (1998) point out that women who have to cover their skin totally, as is the custom for some religious groups, and who are not exposed to sunlight, may experience bone problems because they are unable to synthesize calcium from vitamin D using sunlight as the catalyst.

Likewise Judaism has rules regarding the eating of 'unclean' animal products (which are called not kosher) and eating only foods that have been prepared in a particular way or that have been blessed by authorized individuals. There are also specific rituals concerning washing and dressing.

Nursing care

Routines and rituals associated with personal cleansing bring the nurse into intimate contact with the patient. That which may be perceived as basic or even menial care is in fact fundamental to the patient's sense of well-being, and thus transforms the act of cleansing to an essential aspect of nursing care. Maintaining patient hygiene needs is a clinical skill, the importance of which ranks alongside other skills such as assessing vital signs, administering medication or re-dressing a wound aseptically. In Boxer and Kluge's (2000) research, 83% of respondents rated bathing of patients in bed as an essential clinical nursing skill. It is seen as fundamental to patient care, because it enhances patients' sense of well-being as well as being a functional necessity (Collins and Hampton 2003).

How often patients wash is mainly a matter of personal preference; however, Abbas et al. (2004) write that European and North American women report washing their faces at least twice a day, and bathe or shower once a day. This may become more frequent depending on the weather. Abbas et al. (2004) believe that faces are washed or cleansed more frequently because it is the part of the body that is permanently on view.

Patients prefer to meet their own hygiene needs (Collins and Hampton 2003); however, they value nursing assistance when they are unable to do so (Ratcliffe 1991). This is emphasized in a poem written and published by a patient, severely disabled by multiple sclerosis and unable to speak or hold a pen, about his nurse – Narinder:

I have seen many certificates and diplomas
many gilded trophies too
but only in my mind.

They're for Narinder Kaur
the nurse with elegant hands
and read embossed with truth:
'World record, established September 1990,
for wet shaving, bathing (with hair wash)
and application of gels to gums and teeth

27 minutes.' Signed by me.
So fast were you there was no time for thanks,
so please
may I thank you now?

Ratcliffe (1991)

Helping patients meet their personal needs may be embarrassing for both the nurse and the patient, especially if they are of opposite sexes. Malik (1998) outlines the difficulty male nurses may have in helping female patients, believing that this kind of care is atypical. Female nurses caring for male patients are not perceived to have the same problems because the role is similar to 'mothering'.

Junior or novice nurses may find this kind of care embarrassing, and they may shy away from helping patients with their personal needs. Often it is an aspect of care that has been relegated to the most junior members of staff; however, more experienced nurses find that helping patients with their hygiene needs provides an excellent opportunity to observe the patient, build up working relationships and explore concerns that patients may have.

Assessment

Patients may need help in meeting all or some of their personal hygiene needs, and a great deal depends on their mobility and dexterity as well as their state of health and the prevailing disease. A nursing assessment needs to establish what patients usually do to maintain their personal hygiene, how often they like to wash and at what time of day, and whether they require assistance getting in and out of the bath or shower. A full holistic assessment needs to address whether there are any special needs with regard to cultural observances, so that these practices are not infringed while the patient is in receipt of nursing care. The assessment will include a review of the patient's mobility: can they actually go to a bathroom or do facilities need to be brought to the patient (Malik 1998)?

The assessment should take into account the patient's skin condition, and whether the skin is intact or damaged. Although cleansing the skin removes bacteria, dirt and oil, and is essential and desirable for good skin care, the process could damage the skin barrier, depending on which cleansers are used. Subramanyan (2004) lists several factors that can affect skin and lead to dryness and skin disorders such as atopic dermatitis and xerosis. Stress and anxiety can also affect the skin condition because they may lead to excessive sweating, resulting in increased body odour, which patients may find extremely unpleasant because it can isolate them from close contact with others.

The development of a comprehensive care plan will mean that the patient does not have to repeat the information each time that a nurse wishes to assist him or her in order to meet his or her hygiene needs.

Planning care

Whether the nurse is assisting the patient to meet personal hygiene needs in a designated bathroom or in bed, the operation needs careful planning to ensure maximum privacy, minimum exposure and greatest comfort for the patient. Most patients have with them their own personal items such as flannels/face cloths, towels and toiletries. Some establishments have en suite facilities, but sometimes there may only be one communal bathroom available. The nurse should ensure that this is available, warm and clean before ushering in the patient.

If the patient is too ill to leave the bed, the patient's hygiene needs can be accommodated while in bed. Once again forward planning is of the utmost importance to ensure maximum privacy and minimum exposure. Patients who are ill and confined to bed may well have a 'temperature' and the plastic protective coverings to the pillows and mattress may cause excessive sweating; they may require washing more than once a day to maintain their comfort.

Bed baths

Having ascertained that the patient has consented to being bathed in bed, the nurse needs to ensure that she or he has accumulated all the appropriate equipment – bowl, towels and toiletries. The nurse should make certain that there will be no interruptions during this procedure because it may leave patients in compromised situations that can threaten their dignity and their comfort. The physical environment requires preparation; open windows may cause draughts and chill the patient. Screens that offer sufficient privacy should also be placed around the area. The bed, if fitted with a variable height device, will need raising to the correct height so that the nurse is not bending over and risking back damage while assisting the patient (Aston and Wakefield 1998).

The top layers of bedding are removed, leaving the top sheet covering the patient. Night attire or bedclothes are removed. Most patients will want to wash their own faces, but may require assistance in preparing the facecloth and rinsing it out in clean water before towelling dry. It is very difficult to dry someone else's face; the person being washed is the only one who can feel whether or not the skin is dry, so it is best to facilitate achievement of this task rather than doing it for him or her.

The main aim for the nurse when washing a patient in bed is not to expose too much of the patient at any one time, and to wash the body section by section so that it can be rinsed and dried quickly, thus the patient does not get cold. The water in the bowl will require frequent changing, particularly if the cleansing product or soap lathers up excessively. If cleansing products are not removed adequately, the patient may experience itching and dry skin. Lodén et al. (2003) highlight that mild soap has the potential to irritate and dry the skin if not adequately rinsed off. The soap barrier can build up over time, thus aggravating the situation.

It is usual to wash the upper half of the body first before proceeding to the lower half, and it is usual to leave washing the genital area until last. If patients are able, they will probably wish to wash this area themselves because it may be embarrassing to have this area washed by someone else. It is usual to use disposable cloths for this aspect of the procedure, especially if patients have a urinary catheter in place.

Having washed and dried the patient, the patient may require assistance with applying deodorants, talcum powder, perfume, face creams and moisturizers or make-up before putting on fresh clothing. This is usually a matter of personal preference and the nurse should not assume that the patient does or does not want to use these products. Extravagant use of a patient's products is considered poor practice, especially as some products may be very expensive to purchase.

The patient may be able to sit in a chair for a short period of time while the bed is re-made with clean linen, but if this is not possible the bed is made with the patient still in it. Patients whose hygiene needs are required to be met in bed retain the bowl for future use; if this is not possible, the bowl needs thorough cleaning to prevent cross-infection before returning it to the stock.

Cleansing products

Cleansing products used in washing are largely a matter of personal preference and available finances but may be determined by beliefs and cultural practices. Abbas et al. (2004) point out that soap has been in use since 2500 BC, and that Yardley, launched in 1770, is the oldest brand. However, although soaps are widely used, new cleansers have emerged on the market that clean while not damaging the skin. Some soaps are unacceptable to vegans and vegetarians because they contain animal products such as tallow. These soaps are also often unacceptable in Indian and Middle Eastern countries. Where soaps do not contain tallow, they consist of vegetable oils. Most soaps, however, whether containing animal fats or vegetable oils, are drying and can cause skin irritation, dryness and after-wash tightness.

Most soaps are alkaline whereas the skin pH is slightly acidic; research has been undertaken to determine the extent to which this affects the skin

(Baranda et al. 2002). Abbas et al. (2004) claim that synthetic detergents are significantly milder than soap. Much of the research seems to be driven by public demand for products that are cosmetically pleasing as well as functional. Baranda et al. (2002) discovered that the most highly priced soaps were not necessarily the best; the cheapest soap on the market used in their research was the least irritating to sensitive skins.

Some soaps are being replaced by body wash lotions, which contain emollients as well as perfumes such as aqueous cream. These body washes, according to Abbas et al. (2004), are less drying and the emollients moisturize the skin. They leave fewer deposits on the skin after rinsing and as such do not alter the skin acidity balance.

'Soft towel' bed bath

The 'soft towel' bed bath is a relatively new approach to maintaining patient hygiene that is being practised in some parts of Australia, and research suggests that patients find it more relaxing and pleasant than the traditional bed bath. It appears to take less time, and nurses find it less messy and more rewarding than the traditional method, as reported by Hancock et al. (2000).

Three towels and two disposable cloths are placed in a plastic bag with 30 ml proprietary cleansing lotion specifically manufactured in Australia called Dermalux Soft Towel Lotion. Two litres of hot water are added and the contents are kneaded together so that most of the water is absorbed into the towels. Hancock et al. (2000) do not specify an exact temperature. Malik (1998) describes a similar technique, which stipulates that the water temperature should be 43°C.

The patient has one towel placed over the upper half of the body and a second over the legs. The patient is offered one disposable cloth to wash the face; there is no need to rinse the solution off, and the warmth of the cloth means that there is no need for drying. The upper half of the body is massaged with the wet towel, followed by massage to the legs. The patient is offered the second cloth for cleansing the genitalia. The patient is turned onto the side and the third towel is used to massage the back, ending with the perianal area.

Hancock et al. (2000) report that patients, on the whole, preferred to meet their own hygiene needs, but as this was not always possible, they enjoyed being bathed in this manner and some reported that they preferred it to showering. The nurses involved in this research were also very enthusiastic about the method, because it was quicker, less messy and relatively uncomplicated. Patient satisfaction meant nurses also experienced satisfaction in a procedure completed well.

Using BagBath

Collins and Hampton (2003) outline a new product, BagBath, which is a packet of pre-packed rayon/polyester disposable cloths impregnated with a cleanser that does not require rinsing from the skin surface. The cloths are used once and disposed; there are eight cloths in a packet, so that individual parts of the body are washed a section at a time, maintaining patient privacy. Their evaluation suggests that this is a cost-effective method of providing patient hygiene because it not only reduces time taken to administer but also reduces cross-infection. The use of a cleanser and emollient combined also reduces the risk of 'skin tear' occurring in elderly patients.

Bathing aids

Assisting patients with their hygiene needs may require the use of special aids such as hoists, which help raise the patient in and out of the bath. The hoist may be a frightening piece of equipment for patients, particularly elderly people, because, when the hoist is raised, patients find themselves dangling in mid-air, with little below them as they are swung over and then lowered into the bath. It is important that, while this is done, patients remain covered with towels, and due attention is paid to maintaining their dignity and modesty. The towels may be removed once they are partially lowered into the warm water. It is important to check with patients that the temperature of the water is to their liking before they are lowered into the bath, because this is a matter of personal preference (Switzer 2001). Switzer (2001) advocates that the bath water temperature should not exceed 38°C, as older people may lose their ability to feel the heat of the water; however, allowing a person to test the temperature helps to maintain a sense of control.

There are some specially adapted baths, such as the Parker bath (Malik 1998), with sides that are raised so that the patient can slide in. This makes the hoist redundant. Some baths can be raised and lowered once the patient is in so that the nurse is not bending over and straining his or her back. There are various makes available on the market, and it is advisable to ensure familiarity with equipment before its use with patients.

Hair washing

Hair washing is part of the routine of maintaining personal cleanliness and is a matter of personal preference. Some people wash their hair daily and this is easily managed in a shower. It is possible to wash a patient's hair while he or she remains in bed, but this requires careful planning: it is easily achievable if organized properly.

It is possible to remove the head of the bed on most hospital beds. The bed has to be raised so that the height is comfortable for the nurse to complete the operation without bending over and risking back strain.

There are specially designed bowls available on the market for use in bed, with a spout for drainage. The bed must be protected with plastic sheeting. The amount of warm water required for completion of hair washing depends largely on the thickness and length of hair and how much lather the shampoo produces.

The nurse needs to ensure patient comfort; the rim of the bowl can be softened with the use of towels, and correct positioning is required before the procedure commences. Once the hair is washed and rinsed, it can be towel dried and then blown dry with a hairdryer if the hair is long (Malik 1998).

Mouth care

The mouth is the central and most important part of the face; besides being used for feeding, the main function is in communication. If the health of the oral cavity is compromised both feeding and communication are severely affected (Porter 1994, Henshaw and Calabrese 2001, Rydholm and Strang 2002). Poor oral care may mean that patients experience problems with several activities of living; they may not drink or eat as they would like, and can become malnourished, or they cannot communicate because of dryness (xerostomia), which impacts on their ability to socialize. Rydholm and Strang (2002) found that patients with xerostomia not only complained of the discomfort caused to them from having a dry mouth, but were also more prone to develop infection such as oral thrush and ulceration. They report that patients expressed feelings of shame, which led to social withdrawal as a direct result of this condition. Reduction of saliva results in difficulty with chewing food, swallowing and talking. Finally it makes kissing difficult, which may impact on the patient's ability to express his or her sexuality. All of this reduces the patient's sense of him- or herself and he or she may recoil from the company of others, finding him- or herself isolated at a time when social support is most needed. Listed below are some drugs that may cause xerostomia (McNeill 2000):

Antihypertensives
Anticholinergics
Antihistamines
Antipsychotics
Anorectics
Anticonvulsants
Antineoplastics
Sympathomimetics
Antidepressants
Diuretics

When people are healthy, oral care is a natural part of the personal cleansing routine, and most people brush their teeth at least daily (Paulsson et al. 1999). When ill, there are several factors that compromise a healthy mouth, but generally these may be overlooked as more urgent needs are attended to and given priority by nursing staff. McNeill (2000) points out that, when patients are ill, the normal bacteria in the mouth alter from being

Gram-positive flora to Gram-negative flora, and changes to the oral mucous membranes allow bacteria to adhere, which means that the mouth becomes a source of infection. Nosocomial pneumonia pathogens have been found on dental plaque and oral mucosa of patients in intensive therapy units. There are many other factors that affect the mouth in ill people, e.g. oxygen therapy, intubation, suction, reduced fluid intake. Rydholm and Strang (2002) found that 70% of patients with cancer and 97% of those in the terminal stages of the disease had problems with xerostomia, predominantly caused by opioids and other drugs used to control other symptoms. Previous cancer treatments such as cytotoxic drugs and radiotherapy may have precipitated the condition. Patients with cancer who were interviewed by Rydholm and Strang (2002) stated that they found having a dry mouth woke them up during the night, so their sleep pattern was disturbed; it also affected their sense of taste which meant that they could not cook the meals they previously enjoyed making for friends; in fact, for many, it altered their lifestyle considerably.

Assessment

Several assessment tools have been recommended but it would appear, according to Adams (1996) and McNeill (2000), that few are used as a matter of routine. Eliers et al. (1988) designed a simple scoring system covering the assessment of six categories:

* lips
* tongue
* saliva
* mucous membranes
* gingivae
* teeth.

Nursing management

Paulsson et al. (1999) report that providing oral care is difficult for nursing personnel because the mouth is one of the most intimate of areas which individuals attempt to protect from abuse. A subject in Paulsson et al.'s (1999) research stated:

> One's whole health deteriorates if one doesn't have good oral health.

If a patient is to recover from illness, a good nutritional status must be maintained and this is not possible if the mouth is sore as a result of poor oral hygiene, and aggravated by medication. However, Paulsson et al. (1999) discovered that nurses who were repulsed at the thought of assisting patients with mouth care were less likely to engage in this aspect of nursing care.

They also found that nurses cited lack of time as an important reason for not attending to patients' needs in this regard. Although nurses claim that a healthy mouth is crucial to a patient's well-being, important for their self-esteem, there are those who do not give it the priority that it deserves. This echoes Adams' (1996) and Peate's (1993) earlier research, in which they found that most oral care was delivered by unqualified staff. They also found that qualified nurses were unsure of what should comprise an appropriate assessment, and many were relying on using solutions proven to be detrimental to the health of oral mucosa. McNeill (2000) feels that the reason mouth care receives minimal attention is partly the result of the low priority given to mouth care during nurse training.

Conclusion

This chapter has focused on the need for helping patients to maintain their personal hygiene according to their own preferences, practices and cultural perspectives; this adheres to the NMC's requirements to respect personal preference and individual needs. Maintenance of hygiene is vitally important for the physical, psychological, emotional and social well-being of the patient. It has been deemed 'basic' care, but this undermines the significance and importance that it has for patients unable to meet their own hygiene needs. MacAlister (2001) makes an impassioned plea for this aspect of nursing to receive the recognition that it richly deserves because it constitutes essential patient care.

Not attending to patients' hygiene needs or not doing it well compromises patients' health status when they are already vulnerable because of ill-health, and this is unacceptable when health care is a costly commodity.

Maintaining a patient's hygiene needs is not a luxury but a necessity, if the patient's health status and well-being are to improve.

References

Abbas, S., Weiss Goldberg, J. and Massaro, M. (2004) Personal cleanser technology and clinical performance. Dermatologic Therapy 17: 35–42.

Adams, R. (1996) Qualified nurses lack adequate knowledge related to oral health, resulting in inadequate oral care of patients on medical wards. Journal of Advanced Nursing 24: 552–560.

Ananthapadmanabhan, K.P., Moore, D.J., Subramanyan, K., Misra, M. and Meyer, F. (2004) Cleansing without compromise: the impact of cleansers on the skin barrier and the technology of mild cleansing. Dermatological Therapy 17: 16–25.

Aston, L. and Wakefield, J. (1998) Moving and handling. In: Malik, M., Hall, C. and Howard, D. (eds), Nursing Knowledge and Practice. London: Baillière Tindall, pp. 34–62.

Baranda, L., Gonzàlez-Amaro, R., Torres-Alvarez, B., Alvarez, C. and Ramírez, V. (2002) Correlation between pH and irritant effect of cleansers marketed for dry skin. International Journal of Dermatology 41: 494–499.

Boxer, E. and Kluge, B. (2000) Essential clinical skills for beginning registered nurses. Nurse Education Today 20: 327–335.

Clancy, J. and McVicar, A.J. (1995) Physiology and Anatomy: A homeostatic approach. London: Edward Arnold.

Collins, F. and Hampton, S. (2003) The cost-effective use of BagBath: a new concept in patient hygiene. British Journal of Nursing 12: 984–990.

Eliers, J., Berger, A.M. and Peterson, M.C. (1988) Development, testing and application of the Oral Assessment Guide. Oncology Nursing Forum 15: 325–330.

Ersser, S. and Penzer, R. (2000) Meeting patients' skin care needs: harnessing nursing expertise at an international level. International Nursing Review 47: 167–173.

Gerrish, K. (2000) Researching ethnic diversity in the British NHS: methodological and practical concerns. Journal of Advanced Nursing 31: 918–925.

Hancock, I., Bowman, A. and Prater, D. (2000) The day of the soft towel?: Comparison of the current bed-bathing method with the Soft Towel bed-bathing method. International Journal of Nursing Practice 6: 207–213.

Henshaw, M.M. and Calabrese, J.M. (2001) Oral health and nutrition in the elderly. Nutritional Clinical Care 4: 34–42.

Johnson, A.W. (2004) Overview: fundamental skin care – protecting the barrier. Dermatological Therapy 17: 1–5.

Lewis, K. and Roberts, L. (1998) Skin integrity. In: Malik, M., Hall, C. and Howard, D. (eds), Nursing Knowledge and Practice. London: Baillière Tindall, pp. 247–280.

Lodén, M., Buraczewska, I. and Edlund, E. (2003) The irritation potential and reservoir effect of mild soaps. Contact Dermatitis 49: 91–96.

MacAlister, L.I. (2001) Personal care: basic, simple and dispensable? British Journal of Nursing 10: 1230.

McNeill, H.E. (2000) Biting back at poor oral hygiene. Intensive and Critical Care Nursing 16: 367–372.

Malik, M. (1998) Hygiene. In: Malik, M., Hall, C. and Howard, D. (eds), Nursing Knowledge and Practice. London: Baillière Tindall, pp. 313–343.

Martini, F.H., Ober, W.C., Garrison, C.W., Welch, K. and Hutchings, R.T. (1998) Fundamentals of Anatomy and Physiology, 4th edn. Upper Saddle River, NJ: Prentice Hall International, Inc.

Nursing and Midwifery Council (2002) Code of Professional Conduct. London: NMC.

Paulsson, G., Nederfors, T. and Frdlund, B. (1999) Conceptions of oral health among nurse managers. A qualitative analysis. Journal of Nursing Management 7: 299–306.

Peate, I. (1993) Nurse administered oral hygiene in the hospitalised patient. British Journal of Nursing 2(9): 459–462.

Peto, R. (1998) Infection control. In: Malik, M., Hall, C. and Howard, D. (eds), Nursing Knowledge and Practice. London: Baillière Tindall, pp. 63–99.

Porter, H. (1994) Mouth care in cancer. Nursing Times 90(14): 27–29.

Rassool, G.H. (2000) The crescent and Islam: healing, nursing and the spiritual dimension. Some considerations towards an understanding of the Islamic perspectives on caring. Journal of Advanced Nursing 32: 1476–1484.

Ratcliffe, K. (1991) An Echo of Reflections. Bishops Waltham: Meon Valley Printers.

Rawlings, A.V. (2003) Trends in stratum corneum research and the management of dry skin conditions. International Journal of Cosmetic Science 25: 63–95.

Rees, D. (1997) Death and Bereavement: The psychological, religious and cultural interfaces. London: Whurr Publishers.

Roper, N., Logan, W.W. and Tierney, A.J. (1996) The Elements of Nursing: A model for nursing based on a model of living, 3rd edn. Edinburgh: Churchill Livingstone.

Rydholm, M. and Strang, P. (2002) Physical and psychosocial impact of xerostomia in palliative cancer care: a qualitative interview study. International Journal of Palliative Nursing 8: 318–323.

Subramanyan, K. (2004) Role of mild cleansing in the management of patient skin. Dermatological Therapy 17: 26–34.

Switzer, J. (2001) How to supervise a general bath. Nursing and Residential Care 3: 226–228.

CHAPTER 10

Maintaining body temperature

JERRY LANCASTER

Temperature and metabolism

Temperature taking by the nurse in a hospital or community setting is a common occurrence. By assessing body temperature the nurse can often be alerted to changes in the patient's condition that may have clinical significance, i.e. the patient may have an infection or an inflammatory condition; assessing body temperature is therefore an important nursing activity. Marieb (2004) suggests that body temperature results from a balance between heat production and heat loss. Body temperature is controlled around a set point, which can be altered for a variety of reasons (Pocock and Richards 2004).

To respond effectively to changes in body temperature, the nurse must ensure that he or she measures it accurately; it is also important that the findings are acted on promptly and recorded correctly. According to Dougherty and Lister (2004), there are two reasons why the assessment of body temperature is carried out:

1. To determine the patient's body temperature on admission in order to use this as a baseline for comparison with future measurements.
2. To monitor fluctuations in temperature.

For all forms of life, temperature is a fundamental issue and human beings are no exception. The cellular processes that constitute the metabolism are no more than chemical reactions and how quickly these chemical reactions can happen determine whether or not life is sustained. Temperature influences whether these chemical reactions can occur rapidly enough to produce a metabolic rate that can support life. One of the most important by-products of metabolism is heat, so a simple principle can be applied:

- The higher the temperature, the faster the metabolic rate and the faster the production of more heat.
- The lower the temperature, the slower the metabolic rate and the slower the production of heat.

However, the body temperature of an individual is not only dependent on the rate of heat production; it is the sum total of the balance of heat produced within the body and heat lost from the body to the environment. An extremely hot environment, and anything above the normal body temperature range for humans, which is considered to be between 36.2 and 37.7°C (Higham and Maddex 2001), can add heat and raise body temperature.

The body is split into two thermal zones known as the core temperature and the shell or surface temperature. The core temperature can be up to 9°C higher than the shell temperature and normally remains within the range of 36.2–37.7°C with very little change (Dougherty and Lister 2004).

The tissues comprising the core all have a fast metabolic rate to support their cellular activity and are adversely affected by low temperature. According to Higham and Maddex (2001) the core tissues are:

- the brain and central nervous system
- the organs of the chest, the lungs and heart
- the organs of the abdomen and pelvis, the liver, spleen, pancreas, the gastrointestinal tract and the urinary system.

The shell temperature comprises tissues that do not always require a fast metabolic rate to function because their cells are relatively less active than those of the core tissues, and therefore more tolerant of low temperatures (Childs 2003). The shell temperature is subject to variation with changes in the environmental temperatures. The shell tissues are the skin, the subcutaneous tissues and the fat cells.

The temperature of the large skeletal muscles found in the thigh and calf lies somewhere between the core and shell temperatures. On a very cold day the thigh muscles could be as much as 4°C cooler than the core tissues and the calf muscles cooler by a further 2°C. Table 10.1 shows how temperature readings compare.

Table 10.1 How temperature readings compare

Route	Normal temperature (°C)
Oral	36.5–37.5
Axillary	36–37
Rectal	37–38
Tympanic	36.8–37.8

Factors influencing body temperature

There are many factors that can influence the body temperature. It is important to note the patient's dependence–independence status as well as age. Walker (2003) considers the following factors in detail: physical, psychological, environmental, politicoeconomic and sociocultural.

- Many of the physical factors that influence body temperature are discussed below.
- The nurse must also take into account the effect of a person's psychological state on body temperature. If an individual's psychological state is impaired because of illness, e.g. depression, or affected as a result of medications such as sedatives, he or she may neglect to respond to changes in temperature in the most appropriate manner.
- Extremes of heat in severe winters and extremely warm summers can, as would be expected, have an impact on maintaining body temperature. These environmental issues can be considered in isolation but the nurse should consider the patient in a holistic manner.
- Politicoeconomic factors must also be considered because an indirect factor may have major implications for maintaining an ideal body temperature. The nurse needs to ascertain whether the patient can afford to keep warm – keeping warm costs money. Walker (2003) states that a recommended room temperature for an elderly person is 21°C, compared with 18°C for others.
- It is important for the nurse to note that sociocultural factors may have a role to play in maintaining body temperature. In some cultures there are particular customs regarding clothing, e.g. some women must, as a consequence of religious custom, wear full covering of the body even in extreme heat. Being aware of the social and cultural needs of the patient can help in understanding the needs of a patient in a more meaningful manner.

It is nonsensical to ask 'what is the normal temperature?' and expect to have an exact answer that can be applied to the whole of the human race. Consideration should always be given to the following factors when assessing an individual's temperature:

- Time of day: the body temperature is lowest when the individual is asleep and the metabolic rate is slowest – around 04:00–06:00 hours for day workers. The body temperature is highest between 20:00 and 24:00 hours for day workers. Individuals who work nights may exhibit a different temperature pattern. The temperature differences between these times of day are known as diurnal variation and the temperature of an individual may differ by up to 1°C between these times.
- Exercise or strenuous physical activity can elevate the body temperature significantly.
- Hormonal activity can elevate body temperature.
- Stress and anxiety create responses within the body that increase the metabolic rate and thus elevate the body temperature.
- Ageing tends to lower the body temperature, because metabolic rate declines with age.

- The environment in which the individual is or has recently been and the length of time the individual has been exposed to these conditions affects the body temperature.

Body heat considerations

Production and loss

To balance heat production (thermogenesis) against heat loss (or gain) various events take place inside and outside the body. There are basically five factors that influence heat production within the body and five that influence heat loss from the body. For heat production these are:

1. Basal metabolic rate: the rate of energy consumption in the form of carbohydrates, fat and proteins for an individual just to exist and with no extra activity, such as when an individual is asleep. The higher the basal metabolic rate, the higher the rate of basic heat production; as metabolic rates tend to decline as an individual gets older, so does their resting body temperature (Childs 2003). As heat production relies on increasing the metabolic rate of tissues it is not surprising to find that the remaining four events change metabolic activity in specific tissues or the body as a whole. Where this is achieved by means of chemical agents, the process is known as chemical thermogenesis (Marieb 2004).
2. Raising cellular metabolic rate throughout the body is achieved by the secretion of the hormone thyroxine (also known as T_4) by the thyroid gland. Under the influence of this hormone the cells of the tissues produce more heat because of their elevated metabolic rate.
3. Raising the cellular metabolic rate throughout the body is also achieved by the activity of the immune system and the chemical signalling agents released during the process of inflammation, such as the prostaglandins.
4. The fight or flight response of the body increases the metabolic activity in the brain, heart, skeletal muscles and liver. The chemicals involved are noradrenaline (norepinephrine) from the sympathetic division of the autonomic nervous system (ANS) and adrenaline (epinephrine) itself.
5. Involuntary muscle activity, such as shivering, and voluntary muscle activity, such as exercise, produce heat not only from the increased cellular metabolism of the muscle, but also by friction of the muscle fibres rubbing together (Pocock and Richards 2004).

Heat loss from the body occurs in four main ways: (1) radiation, (2) evaporation, (3) conduction and (4) convection. These processes occur across the surface area presented to the environment, which includes the skin and the upper and lower respiratory tracts. Heat transfer always proceeds from high temperature to low temperature, and evaporation proceeds from high humidity (wet) to low humidity (dry).

- Radiation is the transfer of heat from the surface of one body to another without touching by means of emission of energy from the infrared part of the electromagnetic spectrum, e.g. the heat felt from the sun or a fire. This is the fundamental method by which an individual loses heat from the skin surface; the more skin that is exposed the greater the heat loss.
- Evaporation occurs when there is insufficient surface area for transferring the heat away by radiation; sweat begins to appear on the skin of an individual, and the water of the sweat takes heat from the skin by conduction and is turned into vapour, so the skin is cooled. Heat is also lost by evaporation in the respiratory tract, the heat being lost on exhalation. However, evaporation can contribute to the cooling process only if the water can vaporize into the atmosphere, and so is dependent on the humidity of the air surrounding the individual. Under severe conditions, such as in the desert regions of the world, up to 4 litres an hour of water can be lost from the body through sweating, although the usual daily loss is in the region of 600 ml.
- Conduction of heat is by direct molecular contact, such as the skin molecules to air or water molecules. Under normal circumstances very little heat is lost from the body in this manner; however, heat can be lost very rapidly from the body by conduction such as during immersion in very cold water.
- Convection is similar to conduction; the heat is transferred from the skin molecules to warm the air molecules. These warmed molecules then move away to be replaced by cold molecules and the process of heat loss from the body occurs at an increased rate. It is this replacement of the cold air molecules that causes the body to warm its surroundings until equilibrium of temperature is achieved; thus an individual can lose body heat very rapidly. This is the principle behind the use of fans and the wind chill effect.
- The fifth way in which heat is lost from the body is in urine and faeces, and blood in the case of haemorrhage.

These factors of heat production and loss provide the rationale that underpins nursing interventions related to body temperature.

Temperature regulation

The ability to regulate the internal temperature of the body is known as homeothermy. In the brain there is an integrating centre known as the hypothalamus which coordinates many of the responses required for homeostasis, homeothermy being just one of them.

The hypothalamus receives nerve impulses from specialized cells called thermoreceptors, which are found in the core and shell tissues; it processes these impulses and then sends signals via nerve impulses or hormones to the active tissues to alter the rate of heat production and adjust heat loss as required. Once the temperature adjustment has been made, the thermoreceptor impulses change and the hypothalamus stops its signalling to the active tissues (Marieb 2004); this is an example of a negative feedback system. Activity in the hypothalamus also creates the feelings of cold and warmth, so the conscious behavioural changes such as removing or putting on more clothing may be seen.

In response to the shell being sufficiently cooled, the shell thermoreceptors send impulses to the hypothalamus which coordinates activity with its own cold sensing receptors. The following responses may happen:

- The blood vessels of the skin constrict to decrease heat loss.
- Cellular metabolic rate is increased by noradrenaline (the ANS) and secretion of adrenaline.
- The skeletal muscles begin to shiver to increase heat production.
- Heat loss responses are inhibited.

In response to stimulation of thermoreceptors in the shell and its own warmth sensing receptors the hypothalamus may initiate the following:

- The blood vessels of the skin dilate to increase heat radiation.
- Stimulation of sweat gland activity.

Measuring body temperature

The body measures its own temperature by comparing the activity of core (body) and shell (environment) thermoreceptors. The difference of activity between the two, generating the feeling of warmth, comfort or cold, is shown in Table 10.2.

Table 10.2 Comparison of the activity of core and shell thermoreceptors

Hypothalamus core thermoreceptors, internal temperature (°C)	Shell thermoreceptor, external temperature (°C)	Resultant sensation
Warmth – 37	Warmth – 22	Comfort
Warmth – 37	Hot – 40	Hot
Warmth – 37	Cold – 10	Cold

Thus, it is the temperature difference that gives the individual not only the sensation of relative warmth or coldness and behavioural response, but also the physiological response of shivering or sweating. This can explain why an individual with an elevated temperature complains of feeling cold in a warm room and exhibits shivering, which would not normally happen at that environmental temperature.

The purpose of measuring body temperature is to gain insight into the metabolic activity of the individual, and to monitor the progression of the cause of that change in metabolic activity, e.g. the individual may have an infection, but the elevated temperature is being produced by an increased metabolic rate brought about by the inflammatory response. The same individual could have an elevated temperature after sustaining tissue damage; again the elevation of metabolic rate is brought about by the inflammatory response to clear and repair the damaged tissue, but there need not be any infection.

When measuring the temperature of an individual, it is the core temperature that is the most meaningful with regard to metabolism (Kozier et al. 2004). Unfortunately the core temperature is, by its nature, very difficult to measure. The more convenient measurements of skin temperature are unreliable at best and very inaccurate in cases of low body temperature. The type of thermometer that is available for measuring the temperature also needs to be considered when deciding which site on the body to use for temperature measurement (Johnson and Bouska-Altman 2004). All probes that are inserted into body orifices should either have a disposable cover or be disposable themselves to prevent cross-infection between individuals (Figure 10.1).

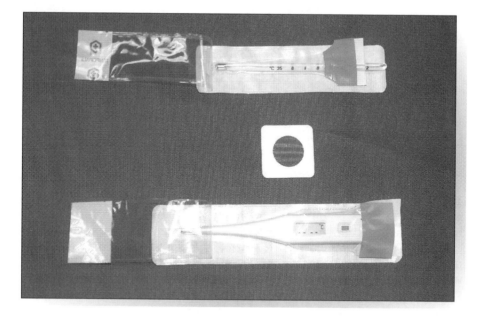

Figure 10.1

Various types of commonly used disposable thermometer covers.

Traditionally, there have been three sites used on the body to assess temperature – oral, axillary and rectal – each site having its own advantages and disadvantages depending on the type of thermometer used. Recently, a fourth site, the tympanic membrane, has become more popular (Kozier et al. 2004). The familiar mercury bulb glass thermometer has given way to the electronic thermal probe for spot temperature measurement which is required for the three traditional sites (Figure 10.2).

Figure 10.2
Various types of thermometer are available to assess temperature: single- and multi-use electronic and glass versions.

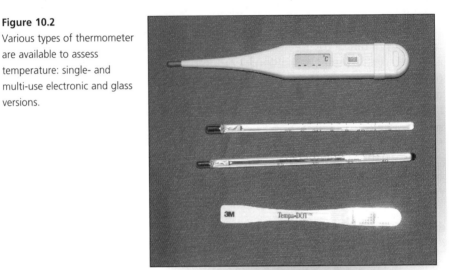

The characteristics of each of the traditional sites for temperature measurement are as follows.

Rectal

The temperature of the rectum, supplied with blood from branches of the mesenteric arteries, is considered to be that of the core; hence, the rectum is the best site for accurate assessment of core temperature. The difficulties in use of this site range from inconvenience and being undignified for individuals having their temperature measured, to inconsistency as a result of the inability to access the same spot within the rectum every time a measurement is made (Kozier et al. 2004). There is also the potential hazard of perforation of the rectum with such an invasive procedure.

Oral

Traditionally the most common site for temperature measurement, the oral site is convenient and has the best chance of some degree of accuracy. The desired site for placement of the thermometer is under the tongue, into the crease made by the base of the tongue and the floor of the mouth. At this site the tissue is heated by blood coming from a branch of the external carotid artery, and so it should provide a reading very close to the core temperature; traditionally estimates have held that temperatures measured at the sublingual site are between 0.5 and 1°C lower than the core temperature. The oral site does offer consistency in the placement of the probe for sequential measurement, but it is vulnerable to inaccuracy, because the time taken for a measurement to be made can exceed the individual's willingness to tolerate any discomfort from the probe under the tongue, and the mouth temperature of an individual can vary as a result of hot or cold drinks, tobacco smoke or mouth breathing. The individual may bite the probe, causing damage to the probe or mouth. The oral site may not be the most convenient to use for an individual because there may be an oxygen mask or endotracheal tube in place.

Axillary

Traditionally this is another convenient site with the least amount of accuracy. The site for probe placement is in the armpit of the individual, so this site is the least invasive; it is not near the oropharynx, so it is not affected by drinking or smoking and does not interfere with the airway. However, individuals can have hollows in their armpits, particularly if the individual is very slender; the probe will then not contact the skin and will register the temperature of the air in the hollow of the armpit (Watson 1998). For the most accurate temperature measurement that this method can yield, the probe must be left in place for a long time when compared with the oral or rectal sites. Traditionally the body temperature measured in the axilla is 1–1.5°C below the core temperature.

The length of time that a thermometer should be left *in situ* at a particular site for the most accurate reading depends on the thermometer type. Electronic probes have their time for optimal temperature measurement preset by manufacturers, which relates to rate of thermal change in the probe, so the user has little choice other than to wait for the thermometer to announce that measurement is complete with a bleep of some sort. Traditional mercury bulb glass thermometers have been the subject of some research as to which length of time produced the most accurate temperature measurement for which site. Traditionally, the optimal time for a thermometer to remain *in situ* for the most accurate axillary temperature was held to be at least 9 minutes; however, not many patients can tolerate a thermometer in their mouth for this length of time and Foss and Farine (2000) suggest that the thermometer should be left in place for 3 minutes. As the mercury bulb glass thermometer was mass produced, the accuracy of an individual thermometer was questionable at best (Fulbrook 1993). These thermometers have ceased to be used routinely in the clinical situation.

Advances in thermometer technology have allowed the use of another site on the body that is reasonably accessible, convenient and potentially very accurate.

Tympanic membrane (eardrum)

The tympanic membrane is supplied by arterial blood from the external carotid artery just as the oral site is; however, the tympanic membrane is not subject to the same factors that can cause inaccuracies of temperature measurement at the oral site (Figure 10.3).

The tympanic thermometer measures the temperature of the tympanic membrane by its infrared radiation; to do this the infrared detector needs to 'see' the tympanic membrane (Figure 10.4). The infrared detector collects the infrared radiation from the tympanic membrane in a fraction of a second, so the temperature measurement is very rapid (Childs 2003).

Figure 10.3
The ear canal and the associated structures.

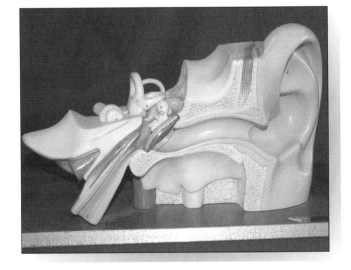

Figure 10.4
An electronic tympanic thermometer. It measures the temperature of the tympanic membrane by its infrared radiation.

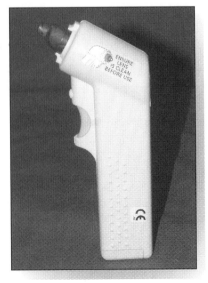

However, this method is not without its disadvantages: the accuracy of the measurement relies on the user's knowledge of the outer ear because the tympanic membrane is difficult to see – at the end of a passage that is at a slight angle to the external ear. Poor positioning of the detector results in measurement of the temperature of the wall of the external auditory passage. If the passage or tympanic membrane is obstructed by ear wax (cerum), a foreign body, excessive hair or infection, the reading may be affected (Gallimore 2004).

It is useful when positioning the probe in the ear to draw the pinna of the outer ear backwards and upwards, which helps to achieve the correct angle for the detector to see the tympanic membrane (Bouska-Altman 2004). Gallimore (2004) cites the following recommendations for practice when using a tympanic thermometer:

- Adequate training for staff.
- Nurses need to use clinical judgement and not rely solely on tympanic thermometer readings.
- The same ear should be used for each reading.
- The same type of model should be used each time.
- The temperature should not be measured using the ear on which a patient has recently being lying.
- The ear canal should be inspected for wax, infection or excessive hair before using a tympanic thermometer.

Chemical thermometers

Chemical thermometers usually rely on a chemical changing colour at a given temperature to produce a reading. There is a tendency for the user to rely on interpretation of the colour change to decide on the value of temperature measured, so the accuracy of these thermometers is questionable. However, they are convenient in use: the strip is easily placed on the forehead of an individual and the liquid crystal thermometer can be placed under the tongue (Figure 10.5).

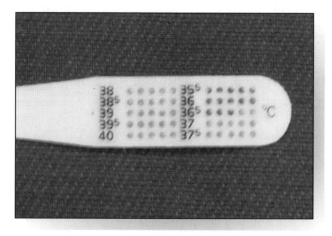

Figure 10.5
Liquid crystal thermometer: convenient to use, the strip is easily placed on the forehead of an individual, or can be placed under the tongue.

Taking the temperature

The method used to assess temperature will dictate how to take the patient's body temperature safely and effectively. Below are some pointers that may help the nurse carry out the procedure competently and with confidence.

The nurse must explain to the patient what he or she is about to do in order to gain consent and cooperation from the patient; explanations can allay fear and anxiety. The patient should refrain from eating or drinking because cold or hot liquids can interfere with circulation and body temperature.

All equipment should be gathered before engaging in the activity because this prevents interruptions during measurement. Privacy may need to be maintained and the nurse must wash his or her hands and, if appropriate, put on gloves before contact with the patient to reduce the transmission of micro-organisms. Disposable sheaths (as appropriate) should be used on any equipment. Electronic equipment should be used as per the manufacturer's instructions. Disposable sheaths should be used for individual patients and should be disposed of after individual use.

After the procedure gloves should be removed and the hands washed again. The reading should be recorded as per hospital policy and in line with the Nursing and Midwifery Council's (NMC 2002) guidelines for records and record keeping. There are four basic body temperature states in which an individual can be; they are the normal range, pyrexia, hyperpyrexia and hypothermia. The following are the characteristic temperature ranges:

- Hypothermia: the core body temperature ranges from 35 to 26°C, with the metabolic rate diminishing to standstill and death between 28 and 26°C.
- Normal temperature range: the core body temperature ranges between 36.2 and 37.7°C. The individual is said to be apyrexial or afebrile.
- Pyrexia: the core body temperature ranges between 37.7 and 40.9°C. The individual is said to have a fever or to be febrile.
- Hyperpyrexia: the core body temperature ranges between 41 and 43°C. At temperatures in excess of 41°C nerve damage is known to occur and at 43°C death occurs. In this range the individual is said to have a high fever.

Extremes of body temperature and the nursing interventions required

Hyperthermia (fever or pyrexia and hyperpyrexia)

There are three basic phases in fever: the onset (chill phase), the course and the crisis (flush or fevervescence phase) (Kozier et al. 2004). The nursing interventions at all stages attempt to monitor and support the physiological changes within the individual's body, ease physical discomfort and pre-empt any complications. Temperature is but one of the vital signs that should be monitored closely throughout a fever.

Onset of fever

The onset of fever is characterized by complaints of feeling cold and shivering (Childs 2003, Kozier et al. 2004). This indicates that the set point of the individual's hypothalamus has been reset to a higher temperature by the chemical mediators of the inflammatory process, known as pyrogens (Pocock and Richards 2004). At this time the individual's body is seeking to raise the core temperature to the new set point.

The nursing interventions at this phase in the fever process would be to provide warmth, but not to excess, and to prevent heat loss while the individual is complaining of feeling cold. Attention to adequate fluid intake and nutrition is required to meet the increased metabolic demand of the individual's body. Measurement of intake and output may be required. Attention to the individual's personal hygiene is very important for the comfort of the individual throughout all three phases of fever. Oral hygiene is required to maintain the moisture of the mucous membranes of the mouth.

Prescribed antipyretic drugs, such as paracetamol, ibuprofen and aspirin, may be given to reset the individual's hypothalamus to a lower set point temperature; this reduces the feeling of being cold.

Course of fever

When the core body temperature reaches the new set point of the hypothalamus, the individual no longer complains of feeling cold. This is evidence that the individual is in the course phase of the fever. The dangers of pyrexia and hyperpyrexia to the individual should not be underestimated; at the higher core temperatures between 40 and 43°C the swelling of the brain known as cerebral oedema may occur with degeneration of the central nervous system, and the kidney tubules undergo tissue death creating renal problems (Marieb 2004). The changes within the brain can be evidenced by irritable behaviour, confusion, stupor, convulsions and coma. The changes within the brain of an individual who has suffered heat stroke may permanently damage the thermoregulatory centre of the hypothalamus, leaving the individual with a legacy of problems in adapting to environmental temperature changes in the future.

The nursing interventions during the course phase of the fever process would be to continue attending to adequate fluid intake and nutrition to meet the continued increased metabolic demand of the individual's body (Johnson et al. 1997). Measurement of intake and output becomes important as a result of increased insensible fluid losses through sweating. Oral hygiene requires more attention to prevent the mucous membranes from drying out as a result of the elevated body temperature and increased rate of fluid loss. Antipyretic drugs continue to be administered and active temperature-lowering interventions need to be employed (Foss and Farine 2000). The use of tepid sponging can increase the rate of heat loss through conduction and evaporation and the careful use of fans can increase the rate of heat loss by convection. It is important that the nurse maintains the patient's dignity at all times throughout these procedures (Nichol et al. 2000). It should be noted that if the temperature-lowering activities are too aggressive the individual's shell can be cooled too quickly, to such an extent that his or her temperature-retaining reflexes are activated; in this instance core body temperature rises contrary to the nursing intent to reduce core body temperature. Provision of dry bedding and clothing are important for maintaining the comfort of the individual.

Crisis of fever

This phase of the fever process occurs when the set point of the hypothalamus is suddenly reduced, and the individual's body activates the heat loss reflexes of dilating the blood vessels of the skin and profuse sweating. The nursing interventions during the crisis phase of the fever process support the continued heat loss from the individual's body and reduce excess heat production. The removal of excess bed linen and use of light clothing help heat loss. Active temperature-lowering interventions of tepid sponging and/or use of fans may continue to be used. In this phase close attention to the individual's personal hygiene and provision of clean, dry bed linen significantly contributes to the comfort of the individual (Kozier et al. 2004).

Not every fever is resolved by a crisis phase; some gradually subside as the stimulus that caused the hypothalamus to raise the set point temperature diminishes steadily.

Hypothermia

At body temperatures in the range 35–26°C, the site of measurement of the body temperature needs to be as close to the core temperature as possible. Traditionally the rectal route is held to be the most accurate site for measuring core temperature in individuals with hypothermia.

The signs of hypothermia that an individual exhibits become progressively more serious with the fall in the core body temperature. As the core body temperature falls from 35 to about 30°C the hypothalamus induces shivering of the skeletal muscles to generate heat; at core temperatures of 34°C and below thought processing and coordination become impaired, and progressive loss of heat leads to the hypothalamic reflexes of heat conservation failing and heat being lost from the core into the shell region of the body. As the body temperature falls lower than 30°C, the heart rate and respiratory effort of the individual diminish, reducing the blood flow to the brain, and the individual becomes very drowsy progressing to comatose. At these low temperatures the heart muscle becomes unstable and susceptible to ventricular fibrillation; pulmonary oedema affects the lungs and the kidneys produce scant urine output.

The intent of the nursing interventions for an individual is simple: to remove the individual from the cold environment and warm the individual's body. However, these interventions must be applied in concert with the individual's heat-retaining and -generating reflexes, otherwise complications may result. Individuals who have a very low body temperature will have constricted the blood vessels of the skin (which gives rise to the pallor associated with being cold); their skin temperature may be much lower than their core temperature. If heat is then rapidly applied to the skin over a wide surface area of their body, in an attempt to warm them up, the resultant reflex is potentially quite harmful.

The thermoreceptors of the skin send impulses to the hypothalamus that the environmental temperature is no longer cold but very warm; this causes the heat loss reflexes to be initiated. The blood vessels of the skin dilate, warm blood from the core flows into the cooler skin and heat is lost to the environment. This causes a sudden heat loss from the core, and as the core cools the hypothalamus still monitors a situation where the environment is warmer than the core. Thus, the heat loss reflexes will still occur as long as the body tissues are at a sufficient temperature to respond. If the temperature continues to decline, eventually muscle tissue will no longer function and vasoconstriction of the skin blood vessels ceases, which may lead to fatal heat loss.

Therefore the choices of interventions to re-warm an individual depend on how cold that particular individual is, and how long that individual has been in the hypothermic state. In all events re-warming should be a steady process seeking to raise the temperature of an individual by 0.5–1.0°C an hour.

The re-warming process of the body may be quite passive, but this would be suitable only for core body temperatures of 34–35°C. Here the individual may be re-warmed by ensuring that the skin is dry and covered with adequate layers of dry clothing or bed clothes; heat-reflective blankets may be used. Warm drinks may be given; blood so warmed, returning from the gastrointestinal tract blood vessels to the core, helps to raise the core temperature. In mountain and cave rescues, warmed air is also administered for breathing, so there is no further possible heat loss from the lungs and any possible cold-induced pulmonary oedema is countered. If the individual is capable of exercising, the skeletal muscles can help to raise the core body temperature.

Active re-warming is required if the individual's core body temperature is below 34°C (Foss and Farine 2000). A core body temperature of between 30 and 34°C is thought to be moderate hypothermia, whereas a core body temperature of lower than 30°C is considered to be severe hypothermia. Active re-warming can be divided into external and internal interventions:

- External re-warming involves the application of heat over the skin surface area by the use of warmed blankets, heat-reflective blankets, heating pads, radiant heat lamps (infrared) and warm baths. If applied too quickly or to excess then the complications of re-warming may occur.

- Internal re-warming: these interventions seek to raise the core temperature in the face of severe hypothermia. Body compartments may be irrigated with warm fluid. The fluids are warmed to above normal core body temperature but below 42°C. This can include warmed intravenous fluids, peritoneal lavage, gastric lavage, oesophageal warming and inhalation of warmed respiratory gases (Foss and Farine 2000).

Any nursing intervention that is applied to an individual with temperature regulatory problems should be evaluated as to how it will work together with the individual's body to restore the core body temperature to its normal range. Each intervention also needs to be continuously evaluated as to its effectiveness and the degree of benefit the individual derives from that intervention; finally each intervention needs to be carefully evaluated for any potential hazard that it might pose for the individual.

Conclusions

In order to care safely and effectively for a patient who has a problem related to the maintenance of body temperature, it is important to have an insight into and understanding of the various complex pathophysiological responses that the body makes when attempting to regulate temperature. The primary aim is to provide comfort to the patient who may have one or several underlying disorders that may impinge on his or her ability to maintain a safe temperature.

This chapter has provided the reader with detailed insight concerning the pathophysiological processes associated with thermoregulation. It was noted that there are several factors that can influence or impinge on the patient's ability to maintain body temperature, i.e. physical, psychological, environmental, politicoeconomic and sociocultural. Being aware of these factors can enhance the quality of care provided to the patient in a hospital or community setting.

The chapter discussed the various methods employed by nurses to assess body temperature. Pointers have been offered that may help the nurse to take the temperature in a safe and effective manner. The nurse is advised to adhere to local policy when carrying out this fundamental nursing skill.

The key role of the nurses is to provide comfort, prevent complications and offer advice. Although temperature taking is often seen as a 'basic' nursing activity, this is an underestimation of the importance of taking, acting on and recording a patient's body temperate competently and confidently.

References

Bouska-Altman, G. (2004) Delmar's Fundamental and Advanced Nursing Skills, 2nd edn. New York: Thompson.

Childs, C. (2003) Temperature control. In: Alexander, M.F., Fawcett, J.N. and Runciman, P.J. (eds), Nursing Practice: Hospital and home. Edinburgh: Churchill Livingstone, pp. 719–735.

Dougherty, L. and Lister, S. (2004) The Royal Marsden Hospital Manual of Clinical Nursing Procedures, 6th edn. Oxford: Blackwell Publishing.

Foss, M. and Farine, T. (2000) Science in Nursing and Health Care. Harlow: Prentice Hall.

Fulbrook, P. (1993) Core temperature measurement in adults: a literature review. Journal of Advanced Nursing 18: 1451–1460.

Gallimore, D. (2004) Reviewing the effectiveness of tympanic thermometers. Nursing Times 100(32): 32–34.

Higham, S. and Maddex, S. (2001) Monitoring vital signs. In: Baillie, L. (ed.), Developing Practical Nursing Skills. London: Arnold, pp. 243–284.

Johnson, G., Hill-Smith, I. and Ellis, C. (1997) The Minor Illness Manual. Oxford: Radcliffe Medical Press.

Johnson, K. and Bouska-Altman, G. (2004) Taking a temperature. In: Bouska-Altman, G. (ed.), Delmar's Fundamental and Advanced Nursing Skills, 2nd edn. New York: Thomson, pp. 29–42.

Kozier, B., Erb, G., Berman, A. and Snyder, S. (eds) (2004) Fundamentals of Nursing: Concepts, processes and practice, 7th edn. Englewood Cliffs, NJ: Prentice Hall.

Marieb, E. (2004) Human Anatomy and Physiology, 6th edn. San Francisco, CA: Addison-Wesley.

Nichol, M., Bavin, C., Bedford-Turner, S., Cronin, P. and Rawlings-Anderson, K. (2000) Essential Nursing Skills. Edinburgh: Mosby.

Nursing and Midwifery Council (2002) Guidelines for Records and Record Keeping. London: NMC.

Pocock, G. and Richards, C.D. (2004) Human Physiology: The basis of medicine, 2nd edn. Oxford: Oxford University Press.

Walker, S. (2003) Controlling body temperature. In: Holland, K., Jenkins, J., Solomon, J. and Whittam, S. (eds), Applying the Roper, Logan and Tierney Model in Practice. Edinburgh: Churchill Livingstone, pp. 257–282.

Watson, R. (1998) Controlling body temperature in adults. Emergency Nurse 6(1): 31–39.

CHAPTER 11

Mobility and movement

IAN PEATE

Every activity of living is associated with movement, e.g. non-verbal communication in the form of facial expression, breathing and the exchange of gases. It is the musculoskeletal system that provides this movement and mobility is an intrinsic aspect of living.

The musculoskeletal system is also responsible for the protection of the internal structures. It supports these structures, e.g. the ribs offer protective support to the lungs and the heart.

The nurse needs to understand the fundamental aspects associated with the musculoskeletal system and how this operates in order to assist and promote the activity of mobility. This chapter outlines how the musculoskeletal system operates to enable an individual to mobilize. It goes on to explore this activity and to provide the nurse with the skills needed to promote effective mobility.

Safe practice

Before moving a patient the nurse must first understand the theories of safe and efficient moving and handling practices in order to prevent any harm to either the patient or him- or herself. The Nursing and Midwifery Council (NMC 2002a) states that the nurse must always act in such a way as to safeguard and promote the interests and well-being of the patient. Wright (1998) states that lifting should be left only to those who are trained in the activity. There is a great deal of local policy that explains and directs nurses with respect to moving and handling, and it is the nurse's responsibility to be aware of these safe handling practices and policies.

The following are useful sources that will help the nurse to practise safely and within the law:

- Health and Safety at Work Act 1974
- Manual Handling Operations Regulations 1992 (amended 1998)

- European directives/guidance on moving and handling
- Royal College of Nursing guidance on safe lifting and handling practices
- Local policy and protocols associated with safe moving and handling within the clinical area.

There are many other sources available that will help to increase understanding of the complexities associated with safe movement and handling, e.g. videos and clinical educators. This understanding will help you to ensure that both you and your patients are safe while moving and handling them. Some types of lift, e.g. the Australian lift, are responsible for more injuries to nurses than any others. The pivot transfer is an extremely dangerous form of moving and handling patients, and can often be seen in use in clinical practice. The so-called 'drag lift' is also considered dangerous to the nurse and patient, with damage to the patient possibly resulting in injury to the upper body muscles and tissues (Holmes 1998). It is therefore important, before moving and handling a patient, that the nurse is confident and competent in these actions that he or she is about to undertake.

The musculoskeletal system: an overview

The presence of joints in the limbs (e.g. the elbow and knee joints) allows movement; without them there would be no movement – the skeleton would be rigid. Cartilage provides a cushion for joints that are exposed to the force generated during movement. Ligaments help to provide joint strength, and either they are incorporated into the joint capsule or they may be independent of it. Movement at the joint is achieved by contraction of the muscles that pass across it (Epstein et al. 2003).

Bone structure

Bone is a collagen-based matrix with minerals laid on it; its strength depends on both components. The mineral aspect is composed primarily of calcium, magnesium and phosphorus. Vitamin D, parathyroid hormone and calcitonin are important factors in bone mineralization (Forbes and Jackson 2003). Bone formation is controlled by osteoblastic and osteoclastic activity, with osteoblasts controlling bone formation and osetoclasts being responsible for bone destruction. Throughout life bone will continue to re-form and re-model itself; it is firm, rigid and elastic (Heath 2000), and dynamic.

The skeleton is the body's supporting framework and there are four types of bone: (1) long, e.g. the femur, (2) short, e.g. tarsal bones, (3) flat, e.g. the ribs and (4) irregular, e.g. the mandible. There are 206 bones in the human body, half of which are in the feet and hands.

Joints

Joints are classified into three types:

1. Those that allow free movement (e.g. diarthrosis)
2. Those that are fixed (e.g. synarthrosis)
3. Those that permit limited movement (amphiarthroses).

Heath (1995) considers four classifications of joints: (1) synostotic, (2) cartilaginous, (3) fibrous and (4) synovial. The synovial joint allows free movement. Bony surfaces are covered by articular cartilage and connected by ligaments. Types of synovial joints include:

* Pivotal joints (e.g. the joint between the humeral radius and the ulna)
* Ball and socket joints (e.g. the hip joint)
* Hinge joints (e.g. the interphalangeal joints of the fingers).

In synovial joints, there is a space between the bone surfaces, which allows movement of one bone against the other. Synovial fluid present in the synovial joint provides nutrition for the articular cartilage and lubrication for the joint surfaces (Epstein et al. 2003).

Muscle

Skeletal muscle has the ability to contract and relax. A motor neuron innervates 100–1000 skeletal muscle fibres and, when contraction of the muscle occurs, the impulse that travels from the nerve to the muscle crosses the neuromuscular junction. The electrical activity causes thin actin-containing filaments to shorten, resulting in contraction of muscle. Removal of this actin-rich stimulus results in relaxation of the muscle.

Muscles are often arranged in pairs associated with two or more bones and a joint. Those muscles that are associated with movement are to be found within the skeletal region, where movement is caused by leverage. The pair of muscles has opposing functions: one of the pair acts as the flexor (contracting and flexing) and the other as the extensor (relaxing and extending) (Roper et al. 1996). The muscles that are attached to the bones provide the necessary force to move an object.

Body mechanics is a term used to incorporate the following coordinated efforts of the musculoskeletal and nervous systems (Heath 2000): to maintain balance, provide posture and ensure body alignment.

There are certain muscles that are associated with posture. According to Heath (2000), these muscles are primarily the muscles of the trunk, neck and back. They converge obliquely at a common tendon, and are short and feather-like in appearance. Working together they provide stability and support body weight, thus allowing a sitting or standing posture to be maintained.

The nervous system

Movement and posture are both regulated by the nervous system. There is an area in the brain (the cerebral cortex) that houses the major voluntary motor area. The specific area in the cerebral cortex - the precentral gyrus or motor strip - sends impulses down the motor strip to the spinal cord during voluntary movement. Muscles are stimulated after various complex neural and chemical activities have taken place and movement occurs.

Movement can be impaired by a variety of disorders that impede the neural and chemical activity taking place. The muscles are not stimulated and movement does not occur. The concept of mobility is complex; there are various texts available that explain this multifaceted activity in more detail. This chapter merely touches on the complexities associated with the activity - mobility. Suffice it to say that, in order to care for a patient with problems related to mobility, the nurse needs to have a sound understanding of the many principles underpinning this activity.

Impaired mobility

Mobility, according to Ismeurt et al. (1991), is the ability to move freely. To mobilize unhindered, the patient needs to engage in both voluntary motor and sensory control of all body regions. The patient needs consciously and unconsciously to notice the sensation achieved through interpretation of spatial position and muscular activity - this is known as proprioception and it gives the patient the ability to move about freely.

There may be many reasons why a patient experiences partial or total loss of mobility, such as the following:

- Enforced bed rest caused by fracture and the application of traction
- The result of paralysis after a stroke (cerebrovascular accident or CVA)
- Postoperative bed rest.

There are several hazards associated with the loss of mobility and the degree of hazard depends on the duration of, and the reason for, immobility. The following outlines some of the physical and psychosocial problems associated with a reduction in mobility (Pellatt 2001):

- Deep vein thrombosis
- Pulmonary embolism
- Increased cardiac workload
- Orthostatic hypotension
- Decreased cardiac output and reduced tissue perfusion
- Chest infection
- Renal calculi
- Incontinence

- Muscle wasting
- Joint contractures
- Loss of self-esteem
- Frustration
- Boredom
- Isolation.

Spray (2003), for example, suggests that patients aged 18–80 years of age, who have been confined to bed rest for an average of 27 days, averaged a 0.9% loss in mineral content per week from their lumbar vertebrae. Bed rest is, therefore, not without its potentially serious complications. The nurse must be aware of these actual and potential complications and be proactive in his or her nursing interventions to prevent or reduce the deleterious consequences of bed rest. According to Day (2004), bed rest can be classed as therapeutic intervention that will help achieve several objectives such as:

- Provide rest for patients who are exhausted
- Decrease the body's oxygen consumption
- Reduce pain and discomfort.

These objectives also link in with the primary roles of the nurse (Roper et al. 1996) to act as a preventive agent, to educate and to provide comfort.

Despite the therapeutic reasons for bed rest it can be counterproductive to the patient's recovery. A number of diseases and conditions can affect the musculoskeletal system during a lifespan – from conception to death (Roper et al. 1996). These diseases and conditions will impair the patient's ability to mobilize. The nurse has a key role to play in helping patients promote independence and to provide them with a sense of well-being (Courtenay 2002).

In certain circumstances the nurse may need to move the patient when he or she is unable to do so. Jamieson et al. (1997) suggest that it may be necessary for one, two or more staff to move a patient using mechanical aids. The following are some of the diseases and conditions that can affect the patient's ability to mobilize:

- Severe injury
- Major surgery
- Paralysis
- An acute illness
- Unconsciousness
- Disability
- Muscular dystrophy
- Osteoarthritis
- Rheumatoid arthritis
- Osteoporosis.

Impaired mobility, e.g. bed rest, can, as has already been stated, result in a number of problems that affect bodily systems. Below, each of the following systems is discussed and the role of the nurse in preventing or minimizing any potential problems is briefly described: gastrointestinal tract, respiratory system, circulatory system, urinary system and musculoskeletal system.

Gastrointestinal tract

The gastrointestinal system can malfunction when the patient's mobility has become impaired, resulting in physical and psychological problems. The nurse must be aware of the potential problems associated with impaired mobility and the effects that this may have on the gastrointestinal tract.

Activity stimulates peristalsis, which may cease if the patient is immobile. When lying supine or in a sitting position the normal reflexes associated with defecation will be absent and this may lead to constipation (Peate 2003). Lack of mobility and changes in diet and intake of fluids may lead to constipation. As the patient is immobile and may be unconscious he or she may have undergone severe changes to his or her usual dietary and fluid intake. If patients are confined to bed they may find it difficult to pour drinks, feed themselves or get up to get their drinks and food, and as such they may reduce their fluid and food intake. Lack of mobility may also cause a loss of appetite. The nurse needs to consider ways in which fluids and food can easily be to hand for the bed-ridden patient. Chapter 8 discusses constipation and the causes of constipation in more detail.

Respiratory system

With immobility there is a reduction in the lung expansion, generalized respiratory muscle weakness and stasis of secretions (Potter and Perry 2003). These changes can result in hypostatic pneumonia (Donnelly 1995). As mucus accumulates, especially when the patient is in the supine position, this provides an ideal medium for bacterial growth and pneumonia may ensue.

The nurse should aim to promote the expansion of the chest and lungs; the outcome will be to prevent stasis of any pulmonary secretions. Change in position will help the patient to expand the dependent lung and mobilize any stagnant pulmonary secretions. The frequency of turning or position change will depend on the patient's condition and a full assessment of his or her needs is required to determine frequency.

Potter and Perry (2003) suggest that the patient who is immobile should be encouraged to have an oral fluid intake of 2000 ml/day, if not contraindicated, in order to ensure that mucociliary clearance occurs. Failure to hydrate the patient adequately will result in the secretions becoming thick and tenacious, and the patient may find it difficult to expectorate these secretions with coughing. The nurse should work with the physiotherapist who may be able to provide chest physiotherapy to loosen the secretions, making it easier for the patient to expectorate them. Deep breathing and coughing exercises may also aid with expectoration; however, the nurse must be aware of the patient's limitations and not over-exert him or her.

Circulatory system

In the patient who is immobilized there is a risk of decreased circulating fluid volume, a pooling of blood in the lower extremities and a decrease in the autonomic response (Potter and Perry 2003). This results in a reduced venous return, a lowered central venous pressure and a drop in blood pressure when the patient stands (McCance and Huether 2002).

Those patients who are immobile are also at risk of developing a deep vein thrombosis (DVT). There are three factors that predispose a patient to a DVT, known as Virchow's triad (Autar 1996):

1. Hypercoagulability of the blood
2. Venous wall damage
3. Stasis of blood flow.

There are other issues that the nurse must be aware of: pressure of the leg on the bed will cause compression of the blood vessels of the calves, resulting in injury to the blood vessel lining and stasis of blood. Normally the calf muscles will aid venous return by pumping blood through the legs back up towards the heart; however, immobility will reduce this important activity.

Stasis of blood will predispose to thrombi formation and put the patient at risk of developing a pulmonary embolism (PE). Small blood clots that have moved from the venous system up towards the lungs are known as pulmonary emboli; they block a portion of the pulmonary arterial system and cause disruption in the blood flow to the lungs (Potter and Perry 2003).

In an attempt to prevent the formation of a DVT or PE the nurse should aim to prevent orthostatic hypotension and thrombus formation. When asking the patient to rise from a lying to a sitting position, or from a sitting to a standing position, the nurse should ask for this to be done gradually, in stages. When encouraging a patient to get up for the first time after a period of immobility, the nurse should also seek the assistance of at least one other person.

The risk of thrombus formation is reduced when therapies such as heparin and elasticated compression stockings are used. The nurse must also ensure that when the patient is sitting there is no undue pressure to the posterior aspect of the knee and the deeper veins in the lower limbs. Patients should be encouraged not to cross their legs, sit for long periods of time or wear tight clothing that could constrict the legs or waist, or put pillows under the knees. An explanation of why the nurse is asking the patient to do this may help him or her understand the benefits.

A range of activities performed actively or passively will help to increase venous return and reduce blood stasis. The patient may be asked to rotate the ankle in a circular motion and to pump the foot as if pressing on a pedal. These exercises should be performed hourly while the patient is awake.

Urinary system

While the patient is lying in the supine position as a result of immobility, this (and the lack of privacy) may make micturition difficult. The nurse needs to be empathetic to the situation, provide a slipper bedpan and ensure privacy when the patient requests or has the desire to micturate.

Urinary stasis may also occur because there will be anatomical changes associated with lying supine; when the patient assumes the upright position gravitational forces encourage a flow of urine from the renal pelvis into the ureter and then into the urinary bladder. Urinary stasis predisposes the patient to urinary tract infection and the formation of renal calculi.

There may be an increase in the excretion of calcium from the skeleton while the patient is immobile. Such an increase in calcium in the bloodstream can lead to the formation of kidney stones (renal calculi), which are stones that are commonly composed of calcium; they can lodge within the renal pelvis and pass through to the ureters.

The essential aspect of care is to ensure that the patient is well hydrated in order to prevent stasis of urine or development of renal calculi or a urinary tract infection. The nurse must monitor fluid intake and output and maintain a fluid balance chart.

Musculoskeletal system

Bed rest or immobility will cause muscle atrophy. Muscles become smaller and their circulation diminishes, which results in a decrease in endurance and rapid fatigue (Donnelly 1995). As the period of immobility increases, the muscle mass will continue to decrease. Joint contracture – characterized by fixation and flexion of a joint – means that there will be a reduction in the amount of movement. Foot-drop contracture can occur, leaving the joint in a non-functional position. Another pathological change that may occur with immobilization is known as osteoporosis, a condition characterized by bone resorption secondary to immobility (Potter and Perry 2003). In this case, the patient may develop pathological fractures that are a result of bone weakness.

Exercise can reduce the damage caused to the musculoskeletal system in the immobile patient and ambulation should be encouraged if the patient's condition allows. However, some patients are unable to mobilize and the nurse may need to perform (with the assistance of the physiotherapist) a range of motion exercises for all immobilized joints, unless they are contraindicated.

___in and the risk of pressure ulcers

The skin is the largest and heaviest organ in the body; it is the primary defence against pathogenic invasion (Doughty 2004). It is a sensory organ and has several physiological functions:

- Excretion of water and salts
- Manufacture of vitamin D
- Screening of ultraviolet rays
- Protection of inner organs
- Temperature regulation
- Sensory awareness of: touch, pressure, heat and cold.

A pressure ulcer or pressure sore is defined as an area of skin and tissue loss caused by prolonged or excessive soft tissue pressure. Pressure ulcers often develop as a result of external pressure which in turn results in occlusion of blood vessels and endothelial damage to the arterioles and microcirculation (Courtenay 2002).

As external pressure is a chief causative factor associated with the development of pressure ulcers, it follows that certain bones that are close to the skin, e.g. the shoulders, elbows, hips, heels and the sacrum, are potential sites for ulcer formation. The pressure sent from the surface of the skin to the bones causes compression of the underlying tissue.

There are certain intrinsic risk factors that may predispose a patient to developing pressure ulcers and these need to be considered by the nurse when conducting a holistic assessment of the patient:

- reduced mobility, or immobility
- sensory impairment
- acute illness
- level of consciousness
- extremes of age
- vascular disease
- severe chronic or terminal illness
- previous history of pressure sore damage
- malnutrition and dehydration.

Although it is noted that there are factors that are intrinsic to the patient, it must also be noted that there are some extrinsic factors that may cause tissue damage and where possible these should be removed or diminished to prevent injury: pressure, shearing and friction. Certain types of medication and moisture to the skin (e.g. in the incontinent patient) can also exacerbate the potential of an individual to develop pressure ulcers.

To prevent or minimize the effects of pressure ulcers, it is an important part of nursing practice to identify those patients who may be at risk of their development. Assessment is the first stage of the process and a pressure ulcer (sore) risk calculator is needed to provide an objective assessment of risk. Risk assessment tools (e.g. the Waterlow Scale) should, however, be used only as an aide memoire and must never replace clinical judgement (NICE 2001). Figure 11.1 describes the Waterlow Scale.

There are many risk assessment tools available and each clinical area will choose the tool that best suits their patients' needs. Timing of the risk assessment should be based on each individual patient, but should be within 6 hours of the start of admission and assessment must be ongoing. The NMC (2002b) states that all aspects of care must be documented; this is also true of the outcome of assessment and reassessment of a patient who may be at risk of developing pressure ulcers.

Skin inspection should be based on the most vulnerable areas of risk for each patient (described above). Other areas should be examined as necessitated by the individual patient's condition. The following may show developing signs of a pressure ulcer and the nurse should be aware of these potential tell-tale indications:

- persistent erythema
- non-blanching hyperaemia
- blisters
- discoloration
- localized heat
- localized oedema
- localized induration.

Those patients who are at risk and have been identified as being at risk through use of a pressure ulcer risk calculator should be re-positioned, and the frequency of the re-positioning will be determined by the results of skin inspection and individual needs as opposed to ritualistic actions (NICE 2001). Re-positioning must take into account other important matters such as the patient's medical condition, comfort and overall plan of care. The aim of re-positioning is to ensure that prolonged pressure on bony prominences is minimized; these prominences are kept from direct contact with each other, and friction and shear damage are minimized. If any manual handling devices are used they should be used correctly following the manufacturer's instructions, because this will help to minimize shearing and friction damage.

The role of the nurse in the prevention of pressure ulcer development is pivotal and he or she is the key health-care professional who should aim to coordinate all aspects of care. There are many adjuncts to help relieve pressure, e.g. circulating air mattresses or waterbeds. Those in wheelchairs may need to have a special cushion applied to the seat of the chair.

If a pressure ulcer develops, the interventions required to manage the ulcer depend on its stage of development and the implementation of local

Build/weight for height	Visual skin type	Continence	Mobility	Sex and age	Appetite
Average 0	Healthy 0	Complete 0	Fully mobile 0	Male 1	Average 0
Above average 2	Tissue paper 1	Occasionally incontinent 1	Restricted/difficult 1	Female 2	Poor 1
Below average 3	Dry 1	Catheter/incontinent of faeces 2	Restless/fidgety 2	14–49 1	Anorectic 2
	Oedematous 1	Doubly incontinent 3	Apathetic 3	50–64 2	
	Clammy 1		Inert/traction 4	65–75 3	
	Discolour 2			75–80 4	
	Broken/spot 3			81+ 5	

Special risk factors:
Poor nutrition, e.g. terminal cachexia 8
Sensory deprivation, e.g. diabetes, paraplegia, CVA 5
High-dose anti-inflammatory or steroid use 3
Smoking 10+ per day 1
Orthopaedic surgery/fracture below waist 3

Assessment value
At risk = 10
High risk = 15
Very high risk = 20

Directions for use:
Assess the patient, circling the number in each category in which the patient fits
Add up all the numbers, including 'special risk factors'
If the total places the patient within the 'at risk' or 'high risk' areas, turn the card over and read the suggested preventive aids listed on the back
Record the circled numbers in the patient's documentation, giving the total and the date
Assess each patient as per protocol

Figure 11.1
The Waterlow Scale.

policies and protocols. The nurse should aim to promote wound healing according to local tissue viability procedures and protocols. Promotion of wound healing will also include the provision of a nutritious diet that is high in protein (if the patient's condition permits) (Courtenay 2002).

Conclusion

Mobility is associated with every activity of living and the degree of mobility/immobility will alter as the patient goes through life – from conception to death. The ability to move about allows us to meet our basic needs, such as eating, drinking and elimination, and also to carry out leisure and work-related activities which will enable us to maintain our social contact and enhance our self-esteem.

Some patients may become totally dependent on others for their care; some may become transiently dependent on others and then return to carrying out their activities of living in an independent manner.

It is vital that the nurse employs the correct techniques for moving and handling patients in order to protect both the patient and him- or herself. There are many statutory and local policies and procedures available to the nurse to ensure that safety is maintained at all times. Techniques for moving and handling patients may be complex but the nurse has to satisfy him- or herself and his or her employing authority that he or she is conversant and competent with these techniques.

No body system is immune to the hazardous effects of immobility; the longer the patient is immobilized the greater the consequences (McCance and Huether 2002). There are many potential complications associated with bed rest that can result in discomfort (physically and psychosocially) for the patient; the nurse has to assume an active role in the prevention or minimization of the potential problems. The role of the nurse is threefold: to comfort, educate and prevent.

Five bodily systems have been discussed in this chapter: the gastrointestinal tract, respiratory system, circulatory system, urinary system and musculoskeletal system. Emphasis has been placed on the assessment of the patient who may be at risk of developing a pressure ulcer and the appropriate care needed to prevent the formation of the pressure ulcer.

The promotion of mobility and helping the patient move from a state of dependence to independence when this is possible are key to preventing the complications discussed. A multidisciplinary approach to minimizing these complications is advocated when this is appropriate.

It is not possible in a chapter of this size to address in depth all concerns associated with mobility and immobility. The nurse is advised to read more detailed texts in order to inform his or her clinical practice and then to develop in more detail his or her clinical nursing skills.

References

Autar, R. (1996) Deep Vein Thrombosis: The silent killer. Salisbury: Quay Books.

Courtenay, M. (2002) Movement and mobility. In: Hogston, R. and Simpson, P.M. (eds), Foundations of Nursing Practice: Making the difference. London: Palgrave, pp. 262–285.

Day, A. (2004) Mobility and biomechanics. In: Daniels, R. (ed.), Nursing Fundamentals: Caring and clinical decision making, 2nd edn. New York: Thompson, pp. 1162–1236.

Donnelly, C. (1995) Care implications for disorders of the locomotor system. In: Peattie, P.I. and Walker, S. (eds), Understanding Nursing Care, 4th edn. Edinburgh: Churchill Livingstone, pp. 351–383.

Doughty, D.B. (2004) Skin integrity and wound healing. In: Daniels, R. (ed.), Nursing Fundamentals: Caring and clinical decision making. New York: Thompson, pp. 1049–1086.

Epstein, O., Perkin, G.D., Cookson, J. and de Bono, D.P. (2003) Clinical Examination. London: Mosby.

Forbes, C.D. and Jackson, W.F. (2003) Clinical Medicine, 3rd edn. London: Mosby.

Heath, H.B.M. (ed.) (1995) Foundations in Nursing Theory and Practice. London: Mosby.

Holmes, D. (1998) Unsafe lifting practice. In: The National Back Pain Association and Royal College of Nursing's Guide to the Handling of Patients. Middlesex: National Back Pain Association, pp. 223–238.

Ismeurt, R.L., Arnold, E.N. and Carson, V.P. (1991) Concepts Fundamental to Nursing, 3rd edn. Philadelphia, PA: Springhouse.

Jamieson, E.M., McCall, J.M., Blythe, R. and Whyte, L.A. (1997) Clinical Nursing Practices, 3rd edn. Edinburgh: Churchill Livingstone.

McCance, K.L. and Huether, S.E. (2002) Pathophysiology: The biologic basis for disease in adults and children, 4th edn. St Louis, MI: Mosby.

National Institute for Clinical Excellence (2001) Pressure Ulcer Risk Assessment and Prevention. London: NICE.

Nursing and Midwifery Council (2002a) Code of Professional Conduct. London: NMC.

Nursing and Midwifery Council (2002b) Guidelines for Records and Records Keeping. London: NMC.

Peate, I. (2003) Nursing role in the management of constipation: use of laxatives. British Journal of Nursing 12: 1130–1136.

Pellatt, G. (2001) Caring for the person with impaired mobility. In: Baille, L. (ed.), Developing Practical Nursing Skills. London: Arnold, pp. 333–359.

Potter, P.A. and Perry, A.G. (2003) Basic Nursing Care: Essentials for practice. St Louis, MI: Mosby.

Roper, N., Logan, W.W. and Tierney, A.J. (1996) The Elements of Nursing: A model for nursing based on a model of living, 4th edn. Edinburgh: Churchill Livingstone.

Spray, M.E. (2003) Care of the patient with a musculoskeletal disorder. In: Kockrow, V. (ed.), Adult Health Nursing, 4th edn. St Louis, MI: Mosby, pp. 102–169.

Wright, B. (1998) Moving and Handling People: Instructors' course notes, 2nd edn. Durham: Training and Learning for Care.

CHAPTER 12
Work and leisure

JACKIE HULSE

Why does a nurse discuss 'occupation', working patterns and leisure interests when admitting or assessing a patient? What are 'work and play'? How can they be affected by illness and accident? These questions are essential to consider before the nurse can offer truly holistic care, and pointers for practice are offered throughout this chapter.

Work is traditionally seen as paid employment, and may occupy more of an individual's time than either sleeping or 'playing', i.e. leisure time. It may provide an income for the individual and dependants, and may often be regarded as a necessity rather than a pleasure! However, work may also confer status, provide social opportunities and enhance an individual's feeling of worth and belonging (Bilton et al. 2002). How often is 'what do you do for a living?' one of the first questions that new acquaintances exchange? Talking informally to a new patient about work or leisure interests may start to build the relationship that is at the centre of care.

It is worth remembering that work may not bring in a salary but be voluntary, or as a home-maker or family carer. It has been determined that, in the UK, some 6 million adults act as unpaid carers for family, friends or neighbours, and that this figure may rise to 13 million by 2010 (Ironside 2004). In 2002, some 12.9 million women were working outside the home, and most of these were full-time workers (Duffield 2002). Thus, the nurse really needs to consider the impact of illness and accident on adults of all ages and not just on the traditional 'breadwinner'.

Leisure time may be seen as that which remains after sleeping and working, and is often jealously guarded. Nowadays, there is an astounding choice of entertainment, activities and travel opportunities available to us in our leisure time. As children may use play to learn and develop, an adult may use leisure time to acquire new skills, enjoy new experiences or simply as an antidote to the perceived stressors of modern life. Work and play may become inextricably linked to health status because an individual may need to work to generate the income to enjoy leisure activities, and clearly needs to enjoy positive health to do so. Similarly, as the range of sporting activities becomes more varied and some activities become extreme, the leisure activities themselves may cause injury or disability that affects an individual's working life.

This simple introduction has therefore suggested that the nurse is asking questions about work and play with the purpose of interpreting any difficulties that may arise from health problems and with the intent of offering appropriate and practical advice where possible. This chapter considers the role and purpose of 'work' in more detail, together with the problems of unemployment.

As identified earlier, work may be paid or unpaid and is traditionally seen to occupy the years from adolescence and/or the end of compulsory education until retirement and consequent eligibility for retirement pension payments. It is worth noting that the retirement age is under constant review by government and a universal retirement age of 65 will be phased in from 2010. This may be a reflection of increased absolute life expectancies and improved health in later years (Evandrou and Falkington 2000), or it may be, as Clarke (2001) discusses, as a result of the perceived financial burden of pensions and health care created by an ageing population. Thus, the nurse needs an awareness of such changes in demography and related social policy for a proper understanding of the situation and expectations of his or her patients.

To 'work for a living' has long been customary in the UK. It developed from offering service or labour in feudal times, through literally working for a living to feed and clothe the family, to working outside the home in the industrialized society. The Victorians introduced 'Poor Relief' and the now notorious workhouses for those unable to support themselves, and this has developed into the systematic provision of state-funded benefits that operates today. Young people in schools and colleges are frequently offered 'work experience' as a taster of adult working life and as part of the important task of choosing a career. Thus, the idea of working to support oneself and dependants is central to our society.

Work provides adults with the means to be financially independent and thus able to make choices about lifestyle. It may even provide a place to live and social activities such as in the armed forces. Paid work will finance leisure activities and hobbies, it may allow for travel and holidays, and it may provide personal transport such as a car. However, work also becomes a much more significant part of the individual's profile and identity. Although the nurse will be mindful of the potential adverse consequences of stereotyping (Eysenck 1996), it may hold true that individuals will choose a career that they feel reflects qualities or interests that are central to their sense of self. Nursing, for example, is consistently associated with a desire to care for people, whereas a hospital technician might focus on an interest in laboratory investigation and scientific measurement. Occupation is used by many governments, including the British government, as one measure of social class. This approach is considered a rather blunt tool and often criticized, but Robinson and Elkan (1999) maintain that such scales are 'a rough guide to the way of life and living standards experienced by the groups and their families'. Certain occupations may be seen as higher status than others and may require a higher level of education and formal qualifications. It is of interest that these occupations may not offer greater financial rewards, although there are still correlations between education and income (Robinson and Elkan 1999). Bilton et al. (2002) remind us that, even if unemployed, we may still define ourselves through our jobs, for example as an unemployed coalminer or out-of-work actress.

Work and the workplace may also provide opportunities for socializing and making friends. Indeed, historically, many large employers perceived a duty to offer welfare and social activities as part of the employment package. Nowadays, opportunities may occur more informally but still remain an important part of being a worker. After all, an employee may spend more of the day with colleagues than with the family. Colleagues may find that the shared interests and aspirations that find them in the same employment are mirrored in common social interests. For those workers who live alone, work may provide invaluable and pleasurable social contact and support. The workplace may also offer support outside the usual circle of family and friends, especially in times of illness or bereavement.

This all assumes that 'work' is a place where a person physically goes on a regular basis, but changes in working patterns mean that this model of work is by no means universal. With the advent of the internet and constant developments in information technology, home working has become increasingly popular (McOrmond 2004) because it is perceived as a way of earning a living and pursuing a career without the complications of leaving one's home. It is seen by many as an ideal way forward for those with children or other domestic responsibilities who might otherwise find their options limited. It means that access to work may be widened for some people such as the physically disabled, who might not have been able to work in some capacities before. However, some of these ways of flexible working are also seen as less secure than more traditional employment, which Naidoo and Wills (2001) suggest may bring other problems; they argue the need for more research into the psychosocial aspects of work in order to be aware of current and future risks. Indeed, not all changes in work patterns are so obviously beneficial to the worker. McOrmond (2004) reports that much work is now non-standard or flexible, which includes greatly increased amounts of shift working to meet the needs of a fast-moving society, and an increase in temporary or casual labour in which the worker may have reduced employment rights.

Gender and ethnicity

It is also worthwhile considering how working patterns may be affected by gender, ethnicity and disability. Bilton et al. (2002) consider that women are still disproportionately represented in jobs such as teaching, catering and retail, which may be regarded as an extension of home life. They also point out that these types of jobs tend to be less lucrative and women's careers tend to progress less rapidly than those of their male counterparts. This is usually attributed to women's role in child-bearing and -rearing and, although many mothers do engage in paid work, this itself may bring other dilemmas. The Joseph Rowntree Foundation produced a study in 2001 that suggested that preschool children of mothers who work full time may do less well at school in the long term than those of 'at-home' mothers. The difficulties are clear to see for the working mother who needs to contribute to the family income, or who, as a lone parent, may be the only earner.

Government statistics present an extremely varied picture of the employment patterns of members of ethnic groups. Parallels are drawn between ethnic minority members and women by Bilton et al. (2002), who say: 'prejudice and discrimination in the labour market lead to the racist equivalent of the glass ceiling experienced by women.' However, Davey Smith et al. (2000) state that 'minority ethnic groups are often concentrated in less favourable locations within a given occupational grade'. This chapter considers *unemployment* and ill health later, but Davey Smith et al. (2000) do present a powerful review of some of the psychological distress and physical problems that may be caused by such inequalities while in employment.

Disability

There is a raft of government legislation (Disability Discrimination Act 1995) to promote equality and opportunity for those with disabilities. Indeed, employers today appear to be proud to display the 'Positive about Disabled People' logo on corporate notepaper. However, as recently as 1998, a large-scale study painted a bleak picture for disabled people in the workplace, including frequent reports of discrimination or unfair treatment and being more commonly employed in lower-paid manual or low-skilled jobs (Institute of Employment Studies 1998).

Unemployment

Having discussed the purpose of work and emerging trends and patterns among the workforce, it is also worth considering the situation of those who cannot work or who work and then become unemployed. Haralambos and Holborn (1995) present an interesting review of the effects of unemployment on the individual and on society itself. These authors highlight studies that suggest that in times of high or rising unemployment:

> . . . divisions within society are likely to grow. The unemployed and those in unsatisfying work may blame weak groups in society for their problem. Immigrants and ethnic minorities may be used as scapegoats with the result that racial tensions increase.

The most immediate and most obvious consequence of unemployment is that of reduced income and potential reliance on state benefits. This reduction in income may affect the food eaten, clothes worn, places visited and so on. If unemployment continues, any savings are used up and real hardship may ensue. As they are subject to change and individual variations, there is little purpose in quoting benefit payment rates here, but suffice to say, as does Clarke (2001), 'that there is no disputing that the unemployed and their dependants suffer considerable financial hardship and material deprivation'.

Health implications

Unemployment

With regard to the effects on health, a study from the Office of Health Economics (1993) suggested links between unemployment and stress and alcohol-related illnesses and mental illness. More recently, Prior (1999) found that a quarter of unemployed men and women reported symptoms such as fatigue, sleep disturbance, and feelings of irritability and worry. According to Peate and Greeno (2001), it appears that men still suffer the most dramatically from unemployment despite the changes in the labour market that have been discussed; they review studies that highlight the increased mortality rates among the unemployed as against comparable groups in employment. Among men, in particular, work may be seen as part of the masculine identity and its lack may cause feelings of uselessness and lack of purpose (Fagin and Little 1984). More recent studies (Pritchard 1992, Stanistreet 1996) have explicitly linked male unemployment to increased rates of suicide.

Thus, if not having work can make you ill, it seems ironic that work itself can also cause illness. We now consider the health problems that may be caused by work.

Employment

Despite the application of well-established health and safety legislation in the UK, the Department of Health (1999) still reported that 20 million working days were lost through work-related ill-health. This may be the result of industrial and occupational accidents or incidents or may be a work-related problem such as stress. The most commonly occurring work-related problems reported by the government (www.statistics.gov.uk) are musculoskeletal disorders, mental ill-health, respiratory diseases, skin diseases, and audiological problems and infections

A nurse may be surprised to read that the same government source reported 251 fatal work injuries in 2001–2002. This was across all industries, and 80 of these deaths occurred in the construction industry alone. As Naidoo and Wills (2001) point out, 'the burden of occupational ill health is not shared evenly between all groups in society' and those who are already economically disadvantaged tend to work in hazardous conditions with less favourable working conditions. Naidoo and Wills (2001) also highlight the changes in patterns of occupational illness that may be expected as work itself changes. Some of these may be positive such as the decline in lung disease suffered by coalminers, but these will be replaced by newer problems. The musculoskeletal disorders best known in manufacturing and industry will be experienced increasingly by those whose work involves the use of a computer keyboard and mouse. Men are currently more likely to suffer a work-related accident but, as women form more and more of the workforce, their risk is obviously increased. It will be helpful for the nurse to ascertain that any patient presenting with a work-related injury is aware of his or her rights and responsibilities under health and safety legislation.

Many nurses will become familiar with Holmes and Rahe's (1967) Social Readjustment Rating Scale and will see that events related to work, such as change in role, in working hours or difficulties with the boss score significantly in heightening stress. A trades union-sponsored study looking at workplace stress revealed that 81% of respondents reported stress as a fairly serious or very serious problem in their workplace (Sparks and Cooper 1997). Nor must we forget that the nursing press carries regular features on stress in nursing itself. In a recent, thorough, literature review of stress, McVicar (2003) concluded that 'workplace stress is having a greater impact on today's workforce' and that 'sources of stress, that is workload, leadership/ management issues, professional conflicts and the emotional demands of caring have been identified by nurses consistently for many years'.

Investigating the links between stress and ill-health is a popular area for researchers in several disciplines. Ogden (1996) summarizes the research that suggests a link between stress and illnesses such as gastric ulcers, heart disease, arthritis, kidney disease and reduced ability to fight infection. Clearly, it is more problematic to determine how much stress is needed over how long a period to cause these problems, but both the causative and the contributory roles of stress seem beyond doubt. The literature on smoking and alcohol consumption offers an interesting insight into the links between stress and changes in behaviour and Ogden (1996) reviews a range of studies that highlight how individuals' consumption of tobacco and alcohol increases in times of perceived stress. Thus, it is useful for the nurse to be aware of indications of stress in her or his patients, and indeed in her- or himself. Occupational health services may be a useful resource for nurses and patients alike. It is commonly possible to 'self-refer', i.e. go along without a GP recommendation, and this service may be able to advise and support before problems become overwhelming. Indeed, in 2003, the Department of Health issued guidelines for occupational health professionals, which urge them to take a more active role in public health and the prevention of coronary heart disease, cancer and mental health problems.

Carers as workers

A relatively neglected group in the literature on work-related ill health are the informal, i.e. non-professional, carers. This is probably because problems are just beginning to emerge as the numbers of carers increase. Wilson (2004) reminds us that the government-driven move from acute to primary care has contributed to this increase, with more people having to depend on family carers. However, as long ago as 1995 the British Medical Association tried to draw attention to the need to support carers. Acting as an informal, unpaid carer is clearly work, yet may bring few of the benefits that we have discussed as being associated with employment. Ironside (2004) states that 20% of these carers are also in full-time employment, which places enormous pressures on them. Those carers who are not in paid work may have given up a lucrative and interesting career in order to take on the care role for a family member. Sale (2004) discusses social isolation and lack of professional support as just two of the factors that lead carers to 'reach breaking point when their own needs . . . impact on their ability to care', whereas Northorne (2000) refers to the existence of the 'overlooked and overworked caregiver'. Sale (2004) points out several extreme and high-profile cases that have resulted in violence by carers and, although she acknowledges that such cases are rare, they have served to highlight the situation of those who are 'caring but not coping'. The nurse will certainly meet many elderly people who are acting as carers for partners of a similar age and needs to be aware of the difficulties that acute or chronic illness can cause to these families. Many carers may be embarrassed to discuss difficulties for fear of feeling that they are failing in the role (Sale 2004), and so the nurse may need to explore these sensitive issues carefully in order to help. At a national level, the government has established a carers' website at www.carers.gov.uk, and a working knowledge of relevant local services and carers' support groups would be invaluable to the nurse.

Illness and accidents at work

For those who are in work, certain illnesses or accidents may have implications for their ability to continue with that work. Those who are self-employed are clearly vulnerable. A self-employed building worker with a tendon injury may not be able to earn for weeks or months and will obviously need urgent advice about his status and right to benefits. A bus driver who has a heart attack may worry that he will not be able to resume his work, and thus anxiety is added to the stress of heart disease and hospitalization. In fact, after a full medical review, the bus driver may well return to work (www.dvla.gov.uk) but the nurse will need to reassure him and his family and he will need to be informed of the process. Some people may not be able to continue in work as a result of disabling illness or accident and some may need to be supported in changing work or roles. It is therefore vital that the nurse is aware of the multiple implications that this may have for the individual and family, and that the patient and family are referred to the agencies that are available to offer support and advice. Nursing itself offers a perfect illustration of this potential problem. Nurses still have to leave work entirely or leave the nursing work of their choice as a result of back injuries (www.rcn.org.uk/resources-wing). As recently as 2003, the National Audit Office published a report that indicated that there were still disappointing levels of accidents and back injuries among NHS staff, with 285 NHS trusts actually reporting an increase in occurrences.

Retirement

Retirement has long been regarded as a significant and transitional event in the lifespan. After a full and rewarding working life, one might assume that people look forward to retirement. Many doubtless do, but this is by no means universal. Bilton et al. (2002) suggest that the pattern is changing and that retirement is not seen as being as bleak as in earlier decades. However, both Clarke (2001) and Bilton et al. (2002) acknowledge the difficulties that some retired people face. These are presented as financial as a result of reduced income and lack of the social identity and activity offered by work. Many white-collar workers may continue to earn in some capacity once retired, but this may not be possible for manual workers. Thus, as Bilton et al. (2002) suggest, 'for less advantaged social classes, retirement may well be accompanied by a sense of social retirement and exclusion'. Interestingly, it is the situation of women that is most likely to change for the better according to Evandrou and Falkington (2000), who report that in this century far more women will be financially better off, having worked to secure their own pension rights. Clarke (2001) suggests that, despite some evidence to the contrary, ill-health is not commonly a consequence of retirement, but may be the reason for it. Indeed, it appears that many retired people even report feeling in better health after retirement.

As discussed earlier, the number of carers in the UK is rising consistently, and so the nurse must remember that, although not in paid work, many retired people provide a vital contribution to family and society. A grandparent may care for her grandchild in order to enable her adult child to earn a living. Thus, any change in that grandparent's health may have an impact on the circumstances of the whole extended family.

Leisure activities

One of the problems that has been identified by carers and the retired is their own isolation and lack of social outlets, and this links to the role of 'play' in maintaining health. 'Play' for adults may be sharing the company of friends or neighbours, learning new skills and so on. Most people might simply regard 'play' as enjoyable time away from work or other responsibilities, but it may also have more concrete links with health status. Indeed, 'social support' has been implicated in helping to improve the experience of those with cancer (Naidoo and Wills 2001) and reducing work-related stress (Ogden 1996), to give just two examples. Clarke (2001) also discusses well-documented links between social support and mental illness, and considers that, although a lack of a social network may not be a cause of mental illness, having a strong social network may have a positive therapeutic effect on those with problems.

However, just as we have considered the ill-health associated with work, it must also be recognized that 'play' may also cause illness and accidents. Ogden (1996) discusses the concept of the 'risky self': an individual whose health is at risk as a result of his or her own apparent choices and behaviour. This is a distinct change from early in the last century when the medical literature largely depicted risks as external ones such as those from a virus, bacterium or water and other environmental pollution. Very obvious examples of this might be involvement in a potentially dangerous yet relatively accessible sport such as skiing. Individuals may consume potentially damaging alcohol or tobacco as part of leisure activities. Although the effects of tobacco consumption may take time to become evident, the problems of alcohol misuse will be familiar to many nurses. This will not just be in the form of alcohol-related disorders such as liver damage but in alcohol-mediated problems such as falls, accidents and even violence and disorder leading to police involvement. There is also evidence that alcohol misuse may play a part in the increase in teenage pregnancies that is being experienced in the UK (Department of Health or DoH 2002a). Of equal concern is the consistently increasing use of illegal drugs as a seemingly integral part of leisure activities for many people. In 2002 the Department of Health reported a national survey that found that 12% of young people had taken drugs in the previous month and 20% had taken them in the previous year (DoH 2002b).

Although deaths of young people from drugs are often reported widely and often amidst sensational headlines, the nurse will also need to consider the effects of drug use among all ages, including the children of parents who may be using drugs, and across all socioeconomic groups. Concern is also rising about the link between drug use and road traffic accidents (DoH 2001), which clearly mirrors the 'drink–drive' dilemmas of previous decades. Illegal drugs are costly and there is incontrovertible evidence (DoH 2001) that links drug use to theft and other criminal activities. Although it is obvious that the nurse may not have the specialist skills needed in this area of care, it is also clear that it is the role of the nurse to offer non-judgemental support and referral to any patients with problems relating to drug or alcohol consumption. Roper et al. (1996) point out the irony which means that something that often begins as a leisure activity may result in loss of employment as a result of absenteeism and poor performance, and they describe the 'deterioration of the self that spills over to affect many other activities of living'.

Conclusion

This chapter has provided the nurse with a great deal of interesting background material when considering 'work and play' for adults. It is clear that, in asking apparently simple questions about employment patterns or leisure interests, the nurse is actually looking at aspects that define the whole person and much about their lives. It is to be hoped that the nurse will be aware of the need to make no assumptions about who is a family breadwinner or about the vital role of a grandparent in maintaining family life. The nurse will need to express understanding of the difficulties and even despair faced by those without work or by those who seem pressured to return to work despite poor health. Nursing care will be most successful if offered in partnership with the patient and family, and this partnership will result only from a thorough understanding and acceptance of the patient and his or her situation in life.

References

Bilton, T., Bonnet, K., Jones, P. et al. (2002) Introductory Sociology, 4th edn. Basingstoke: Palgrave.

British Medical Association (1995) Taking Care of the Carers. London: BMJ Books.

Clarke, A. (2001) The Sociology of Healthcare. Harlow: Pearson Education.

Davey Smith, G., Charsley, K., Lambert, L., Paul, S., Fenton, P. and Ahmad, W. (2000) Ethnicity, health and the meaning of socio-economic position. In: Graham, H. (ed.), Understanding Health Inequalities. Milton Keynes: Open University Press, chapter 2.

Department of Health (1999) Our Healthier Nation. London: DoH.

Department of Health (2001) Report to the Advisory Council on the Misuse of Drugs. London: DoH.

Department of Health (2002a) National Alcohol Harm Reduction Strategy. London: DoH.

Department of Health (2002b) Young People and Drug Misuse. London: DoH.

Department of Health (2003) Taking a Public Health Approach in the Workplace. London: DoH.

Duffield, M. (2002) Trends in female employment. Labour Market Trends 110: 11.

Evandrou, M. and Falkington, J. (2000) Looking back to look forward; lessons from four birth cohorts in the twenty first century. Population Trends 99: 10.

Eysenck, M. (1996) Simply Psychology. Hove: Psychology Press.

Fagin, L. and Little, M. (1984) The Forsaken Families. Harmondsworth: Penguin.

Haralambos, M. and Holborn, M. (1995) Sociology Themes and Perspectives, 4th edn. London: Unwin Hyman.

Holmes, T. and Rahe, R. (1967) The social readjustment rating scale. Journal of Psychosomatic Research 11: 213–218.

Institute of Employment Studies (1998) Employment of disabled people: assessing the extent of participation. London: IES.

Ironside, V. (2004) Just give me a break. The Times 3 April: 6.

Joseph Rowntree Foundation (2001) Full time work by parents of under fives and links to risks of lower attainment by children. London: Joseph Rowntree (www.jrf.org.uk).

McOrmond, T. (2004) Changes in working trends over the last decade. Labour Market Trends Jan.: 25–34.

McVicar, A. (2003) Workplace stress: a literature review. Journal of Advanced Nursing 44: 633–642.

Naidoo, J. and Wills, J. (2001) Health Studies: An introduction. Basingstoke: Palgrave.

National Audit Office (2003) A Safer Place to Work. London: HMSO.

Northorne, L. (2000) The overlooked and overworked caregiver. Social Science and Medicine 50: 271–284.

Office of Health Economics (1993) The Impact of Unemployment on Health. London: OHE.

Ogden, J. (1996) Health Psychology: A textbook. Milton Keynes: Open University Press.

Peate, I. and Greeno, M. (2001) The consequences of male unemployment. Practice Nursing 12: 460–462.

Prior, P. (1999) Gender and Mental Health. London: Macmillan.

Pritchard, C. (1992) Is there a link between suicide in young men and unemployment? A comparison of the UK with other European Community countries. British Journal of Psychiatry 160: 750–756.

Robinson, J. and Elkan, R. (1999) Health Needs Assessment: Theory and practice. London: Churchill Livingstone.

Roper, N., Logan, W. and Tierney, A. (1996) The Elements of Nursing, 4th edn. Edinburgh: Churchill Livingstone.

Sale, A. (2004) Caring but not coping. Community Care 29: 32–33.

Sparks, K. and Cooper, C. (1997) Occupational awareness and response to workplace stress: survey of TGWU health and safety representatives. Manchester: UMIST.

Stanistreet, D. (1996) Injury and poisoning mortality amongst young men. Working with Men 3: 16–18.

Wilson, V. (2004) Supporting family carers in the community setting. Nursing Standard 18(9): 47–55.

CHAPTER 13

Human sexuality and sexual health

IAN PEATE

Human sexuality is a diverse subject and nurses will need to consider it if they are to provide holistic care. The care that the nurse provides must be based on and around the tenets of the *Code of Professional Conduct* (Nursing and Midwifery Council [NMC] 2002) in order to respect the patient or client as an individual. Sex and sexuality are central to what humans are. Hence, nurses are in danger of ignoring a large aspect of the patient's being if they ignore his or her sexuality and any issues surrounding his or her sexual health needs.

Health-care professionals have had and may still be experiencing difficulty in attempting to find a definition that captures the true essence of what it is to be a sexual being (White and Heath 2002). The World Health Organization (1986) suggests that sexuality and sexual health are made up of three chief components:

1. A capacity to enjoy and control sexual and reproductive behaviour in accordance with a social and personal ethic.
2. Freedom from psychological factors such as fear, shame, guilt and false beliefs inhibiting the sexual response and impairing sexual relationships.
3. Freedom from organic disease, disorders and deficiencies that impair sexual and reproductive functioning.

This definition points to the fact that the concept of sexuality encompasses more than sex as a basic sex need; it includes consideration of aspects of the individual from a physical, psychological and social perspective. Sexual health has also been defined by Greenhouse (1994) as: 'Enjoyment of sexual activity of one's choice, without causing or suffering physical or mental harm.' Illness, chronic conditions and hospitalization can affect sexuality; according to Webb (1985) this can also impact on the individual's ability to enjoy the sexual activity of their choice. Sexual health is an important part of mental and physical health (Department of Health [DoH] 2001).

Expressions of sexuality

Individuals need to be able to express their desired sexuality in whatever way they feel comfortable. Early work from the 1940s and 1950s, e.g. Kinsey et al. (1948, 1953), describes a continuum of human sexuality, suggesting that homosexuality and heterosexuality are not necessarily exclusive represent-ations for a lot of people.

Nurses work with patients in a clinical, therapeutic context and they can find themselves getting close to the patient in terms of being privileged to learn about the patient's sexuality. Nurses have the potential to help and educate patients by listening, talking and supporting. The way nurses respond to their patients' sexual identities as they wish to express them can either help or hinder individuals' expressions of sexuality. Nurses are also sexual beings and as such each nurse has her or his own sense of identity, and sense of sexual identity. The sexual identity of the nurse as well as that of the patient will develop and change. Wells (2000) states that when addressing the sexual needs of the patient the nurse may feel as if she or he is taking steps into the unknown. Taking these first steps may be difficult but, if the nurse is to act in the patient's best interests, this has to happen. The important thing is for the nurse to understand that this feeling is usual and, with practice and preparation, the feelings will subside and addressing the important issue of sexuality will become a usual part of the assessment process.

Sexual identity develops as we age and is not to be seen as something with which individuals are born; instead it develops through experience and, because of this, sexual identity has social significance and is subject to social understanding (Weeks 1993). There are three components of sexual identity according to Ingram-Fogel (1990): biological sex, gender identity and gender role orientation.

Biological sex refers to a person's chromosomal make-up, external genitalia, hormonal states and secondary sexual characteristics. It is during conception that the process of sexual differentiation begins. In the prenatal period anomalies related to sexual development can occur, but it is not until birth that an individual can be said to have a sexual identity. After birth and in later life sexual anomalies can present.

For an individual to develop an adequate sexual identity he or she must conform to certain sex-typed norms. Associated with sexual identity is the notion of gender identity. Gender identity is linked to an individual's belief of being male or female and as such he or she is aware of the self as either male or female.

Gender or sex role orientation refers to learning or performing the accepted characteristics and behaviours for a given sex; little boys learn what big boys do and little girls learn what big girls do. Society determines what the socially accepted characteristics and behaviours are for each given sex. This can influence the way a nurse cares for patients, e.g. if he or she draws on past experiences; likewise the nurse must also be aware that the patient may be drawing on his or her own personal platform in order to address his or her sexual needs.

Communicating with patients about sexuality

Many people find talking about intimate topics such as sexuality difficult or problematic; this is also true in the nurse–patient relationship. Sexual health problems can be presented to the nurse in a variety of ways: sometimes indirect and sometimes covert. Nurses are often faced with or have the opportunity to address sexuality in various health-care settings, e.g. community/primary care venues, occupational health locations, the prison service and maternity settings.

Chapter 4 is concerned with the nursing skill of communication. Communication skills can be continually improved upon and the nurse needs to develop and enhance them very early on in his or her professional career. In this section the aim is to encourage the nurse to address and begin to make inroads when talking to patients about sex and sexuality. Health-care professionals vary concerning the degree of ease and comfort that they express when discussing sexuality with patients. Curtis et al. (1995) point out that some nurses might fear that patients may feel that sexual health does not fall within their remit or that it is intrusive to be asked about sexual activity. These fears, suggest Curtis et al. (1995), may be misplaced, because often patients regard it as appropriate for nurses to enquire about sexual health when assessing such needs.

Taking a sexual health history

When assessing a patient's individual needs the nurse must also consider sexual health needs. Chapter 2 describes the general assessment process in detail; this section concentrates on how to take a sexual health history confidently, in order to assess the patient's needs fully.

It has been stated that gathering data from a patient in order to obtain a comprehensive sexual health history can be somewhat intimidating for some nurses. There are ways in which the anxiety associated with this process can be alleviated. Understanding of the reason for taking the sexual health history may reduce anxiety. It is also important for the nurse to know that the patient may be feeling ill at ease. The overall aim for taking the sexual health history is to allow the patient to communicate with the nurse about his or her sexual worries. It is important, therefore, that the nurse makes the environment in which the history taking is to take place as non-threatening an environment as possible, to encourage the patient to speak about his or her concerns.

The nurse should aim to avoid some of the potential barriers to effective sexual health history taking. Often nurses are busy and this in itself can be seen as a barrier to taking a good in-depth sexual history. Managing time is an essential skill that can ensure that the activity runs smoothly. Lack of knowledge can also hinder the successful taking of a sexual health history, but the nurse has a duty to maintain professional knowledge and competence (NMC 2002). The nurse must also recognize his or her limitations and where his or her professional boundaries are, in order to refer the patient to a more appropriate agency, e.g. a sexual health adviser. The NMC (2002) states that nurses must acknowledge any limits associated with their professional competence.

Communication is a key skill that the nurse needs to possess and develop; often patients may use 'street talk' in order to explain their needs. It is vital that the nurse is continually 'checking out' what he or she thinks the patient means in order to avoid confusion. Misinterpretation of important issues can lead to dire consequences and can be disastrous for patient care. Once the nurse has developed his or her repertoire of 'street talk', using this mode of communication will become easier for both patient and nurse.

A key barrier to taking a sexual health history successfully can be embarrassment (Jewitt 1995). Acknowledgement that the role of the nurse in assessing a patient's holistic health status will include assessment of their sexual health may alleviate feelings of embarrassment. Table 13.1 outlines some of the potential barriers to taking an effective sexual health history.

Table 13.1 Potential barriers to effective sexual history taking

Time	The management of time is paramount. Sexual health and history taking require much time and consideration
Knowledge base	Lack of knowledge on both patient's and nurse's behalf. The nurse needs to ensure that his or her knowledge base is up to date and complete
Communication skills	With every consultation effective communication skills are very important. It is possible for misinterpretation to occur and care must be taken to prevent this. Ask for clarification of 'street talk' if needed
Fear	Dealing with complex, sensitive and sometimes legally bounded issues such as rape may be problematic. It is important that the nurse understands that she or he will not be expected to be able to cope with all the issues raised during the consultation. Appropriate referral may be needed
Interruptions	Interruptions by other health-care professionals or by the telephone can often impinge on the sexual health history taking activity. The nurse should be aware that the patient is less likely to divulge important information if he or she fears being overheard. It is important for the nurse to ensure that interruptions do not occur and that the risk of being overheard is minimized

Adapted from Peate (1997).

The nurse should ask appropriate questions, and the patient also needs to know that the questions being asked are valid, i.e. justifiable and necessary. The types of questions being asked by the nurse may be seen as socially unacceptable, e.g. personal questions such as 'what type of sexual activity does the patient engage in?' (Jewitt 1995). However, if the nurse explains clearly the reasons for asking such questions, this may ease the way in which the consultation progresses.

When the consultation begins the nurse should begin by asking open-ended questions and then proceed to more complex and more personal types of questions. The nurse may choose to use medical terminology and/or 'street talk'; this does not matter as long as both the patient and the nurse do not misunderstand each other. Questions should be asked in a clear, unambiguous and, most importantly, non-judgemental manner. The role of the nurse is varied and multifaceted; it is not, however, the role of the nurse to cast judgement on the patient or his or her sexual preferences. Here is a list of suggested strategies that may enhance the sexual health history-taking process (Jewitt 1995):

- A pleasant environment for the consultation
- Privacy
- Freedom from interruptions
- A quiet environment
- Positioning of furniture – spatial distancing
- The less clinical the environment, the better
- Sufficient material resources
- Be aware of verbal and non-verbal communications
- Appropriate language, e.g. medical and/or street talk
- Respect for the patient
- Focus on the patient's needs
- Ask focused questions
- Sensitivity and empathy
- Empower the patient
- Do not make any assumptions
- Avoid stereotyping the patient.

The nurse is ideally placed to assess a patient's sexual health needs by taking a sexual health history. Nurses should be encouraged to take up existing opportunities in order to address sexual health issues with patients. It is important when assessing sexual health needs that the nurse be aware of the patient's feelings, e.g. embarrassment or fear. Recommendations for good practice include the following:

- Nurses should take the opportunity to assess sexual health needs as they would assess any other needs that the patient may have.
- In order to provide the patient with the correct sexual health advice, the nurse needs to ensure that his or her knowledge base is up to date.

- The nurse can provide the patient with information in a variety of ways and this may include the use of leaflets, posters and electronic media.
- Effective communication skills are vital if the nurse is to encourage the patient to divulge sensitive information.
- Being aware of local referral agencies will help to promote appropriate referrals.

There are several ways in which the services offered to people with sexual health difficulties can be improved; the following outline some ways of improving the experience that the patient may encounter when accessing sexual health services (Wakely 2001):

- Try not to make assumptions about a patient when taking a sexual health history, e.g. it is better to talk to patients about their partners as opposed to their wives or girlfriends, their husbands or boyfriends.
- Give a patient permission to divulge sensitive information, i.e. do not employ a judgemental attitude.
- Try to use patient education materials that emphasize that any information the patient discloses will be treated with respect and dealt with in confidence.
- Be aware of appropriate referral agencies.

The effect that illness may have on an individual's sexuality

Illness in its various forms can be transient, i.e. acute, or persistent, i.e. chronic; no matter what the outcome for the person, this can have significant consequences for his or her sexual health. The result of the illness may impinge on the person's self-concept, the individual's body image, e.g. the loss of a body part, and the ability to live a life independently and with a degree of privacy. Some illnesses may mean that the person has to depend on others in order to carry out some of the activities of living, e.g. washing and bathing. The illness itself may also cause the patient potential problems, e.g.

- reduction/loss of mobility
- shortness of breath
- musculoskeletal problems, e.g. osteoarthritis
- sexually transmitted infections
- lack of energy
- dementia
- effects of Parkinson's disease, e.g. muscular rigidity.

Body image

Knowing that he or she is sexually attractive to others can be an important boost to an individual's self-esteem. However, when the individual's self-esteem associated with body image is flawed, e.g. by surgical intervention, injury or illness, he or she may have low self-esteem and the subsequent things that this brings with it (Rutter 2000). Conflict between body reality and body ideal can result in altered body image.

Ageing

Age-related changes can also impinge on body image; as people age, their bodies undergo transitions. The physically related changes that occur as a person ages can influence how he or she feels about him- or herself. He or she may feel differently as a sexual being, feel less attractive, less desirable or less useful.

Normal changes that occur as the body ages can have an effect on the physical act of sex – sexual functioning. This may lead to feelings of frustration, anxiety and fear. The outcome of these feelings can result in the individual stopping or limiting sexual activity. Men and women might experience different age-related changes. Women may, because of oestrogen diminution, have vaginal dryness and/or less orgasmic sensation. The older man may experience changes in erectile function and there may also be changes in his ability to ejaculate. It is, however, important to note that the pathological causes associated with altered sexual functioning can occur at any age (Riley 1999), although these pathological causes appear to occur more commonly in advancing years.

People with real or in some cases imagined body loss have the same sexual needs as any other person and nurses must ensure that the care they provide does not deny the patient these sexual needs. Relationships, e.g. the relationship between a husband and his wife, can be altered during a phase of hospitalization. The relationship between these two individuals can change; they may no longer (albeit temporarily) be able to interact or be intimate with each other. The nurse has the ability to help the patient adjust to this change.

Mastectomy

A positive approach is required when caring for the patient with altered body image – such as following a mastectomy. The nurse should strive to encourage the patient to remain in control, to encourage independence and to take part in the decision-making process. The nurse will need to assume the role of listener and counsellor to both the patient and the patient's family. For those patients who have undergone mastectomy, they may be experiencing problems associated with alterations in sexuality and sexual expression; the patient should be encouraged to speak openly about anxieties and fears.

For many women who undergo mastectomy as a result of breast cancer, it is estimated that at least one in three will experience sexual difficulties a year after mastectomy (Smeltzer and Bare 2000). Some women may find it difficult to look at the operation site after a mastectomy; encouraging the woman and her partner to explore feelings may reduce stress and anxiety. The nurse can offer the woman practical advice about sexual concerns, e.g. that the woman and her partner vary the time of day they engage in sexual activity (when the woman feels less tired), to assume positions with which the woman feels comfortable and also to reiterate that expressions of sexuality can be done in many other ways, not just sexual intercourse. The number of men who have undergone mastectomy and the effects that this has on their sexual experiences after a mastectomy are yet to be established.

Formation of colostomy or ileostomy

Often a colostomy or ileostomy is performed because the patient has cancer; as with breast cancer patients, the nurse needs to be sensitive and to develop his or her listening skills. Preoperative information must be given in such a way that the patient is able to make an informed decision about surgery and the potential effects that this might have on them, e.g. potential damage to nerves may result in failure of erection.

Often patients view surgical intervention as mutilating and, as such, a threat to their sexuality. The presence of a colostomy/ileostomy appliance should be no bar to sexual activity; however, the appliance itself may be a cause of anxiety. Specifically, the patient may need to be told about techniques that can be used during intercourse to reduce any anxieties. Practical advice will include emptying the appliance before sexual activity, and taping the appliance to the abdominal wall in order to reduce its interference with the sex act. Positions may need to be altered in order to reduce pressure on the abdomen or tender scar tissue, e.g. the 'spoons' position.

Removal of the rectum is necessary in some surgical cases and this may cause distress in those patients who engage in anal intercourse. In this case the nurse needs to listen to anxieties and fears, respect the individual, be non-judgemental and, if appropriate, suggest alternative methods of enjoying and expressing sexuality.

Hysterectomy

The uterus is often associated with a woman's self-concept of herself. After a hysterectomy the woman will no longer menstruate and she may feel that her perception of herself as a female has been breached. A consequence of this might be a reduction in self-esteem and self-image; she may feel less sexually desirable. Rutter (2000) states that some women may have been misinformed about the operation itself and the myth may abound which suggests that during the removal of the uterus the vagina is 'sewn up'. It is therefore paramount that information given preoperatively should be detailed and accessible; before the woman gives informed consent to the procedure the woman should be given as much information as possible in order to truly understand the potential implications of surgery, e.g. potential nerve damage and scar tissue formation, possibly resulting in decreased genital sensitivity. The following details some issues that may need to be discussed with the woman preoperatively (de Marquiegui and Huish 1999):

- Explain the potential risks to sexuality
- Encourage the woman to express fears and address myths
- Assist in communication between partners (if appropriate)
- Reinforce the fact that genital sex is not the only form of sexual expression
- Explore and discuss other forms of sexual intimacy
- Be prepared to offer alternative forms of support, e.g. referral to other agencies.

It needs to be explained sensitively to the woman that the pain and tenderness she is feeling postoperatively will subside and that she will be able to resume sexual activity as soon as she feels comfortable. The nurse can advise the woman that she may need to alter position during or before sexual intercourse in order to reduce abdominal or vaginal discomfort.

Preoperative information giving might also include information for the woman's partner. Cairns (1983) explains that about 50% of men go on to develop secondary impotence after their partners have undergone a hysterectomy. The nurse, therefore, as part of the sexual rehabilitative process, should consider giving information to the woman's partner.

Coronary heart disease

A life-threatening event such as myocardial infarction can often instil feelings of fear and anxiety in patients about the resumption of 'normal' activity. This anxiety and fear can also be problematic when the individual begins to contemplate the resumption of sexual activity – whatever that type of sexual activity might be.

It could be that the patient and/or the partner may have fears of death during sexual intercourse. However, this is rare and Wakely (2001) suggests that only 0.6% of sudden deaths occur during intercourse. The fear of inciting an attack of angina may also be felt by either the patient or the partner. In both instances the nurse should be prepared to sit and talk through the fears and anxieties that the patient may have. Explanation of the risks to the patient may reduce anxiety and fears. The nurse should also remind the patient about taking any angina prophylaxis medications before engaging in what may be seen as a stressful event, i.e. sexual intercourse. It might also help to reduce the physical burden of sexual activity if the patient's partner assumes a more active role during sexual intercourse.

For some people who have experienced and survived a myocardial infarction, their quality of life and subsequently the quality of their sex life may be affected psychologically as well as physically. Self-confidence can take a serious blow and the fear of another 'heart attack' may be on the patient's mind, especially in the early months after the myocardial infarction. By being aware and offering the patient advice and support, the nurse can help to rebuild and strengthen self-confidence.

Injury, e.g. facial disfigurement

The result of trauma, e.g. a road traffic accident, or the presence of a congenital deformity can leave the patient facially and psychologically disfigured. The nurse has to help the individual come to terms with a variety of emotions and feelings. Helping the patient is a huge challenge because the facial disfigurement is likely to result in complications associated with social, intimate and sexual relationships (Roberts 2000). The role of the nurse is to attempt to create an atmosphere that is open and honest and to encourage the patient to become a part of society again, to re-establish, as far as possible, his or her previous lifestyle. The key skill is to be honest with the person and to refer the patient when the nurse has acknowledged his or her limitations. Partridge (1994) provides a model (the scared syndrome) that outlines how facially disfigured and non-facially disfigured people behave during social contact (Table 13.2).

Table 13.2 The scared syndrome

You			They	
Feel	Behave		Behave	Feel
Self-conscious	Submissive	S	Staring	Sympathy
Conspicuous	Clumsy	C	Curiosity	Caution
Angry	Apathy	A	Awkwardness	Anguished
Resentful	Regressive	R	Rudeness	Reluctant
Empty	Excluded	E	Evasiveness	Embarrassed
Different	Defenceless	D	Distance	Dread

From Partridge (1994).

Stigma

Goffman (1963) discusses the effects of stigma on individuals. Stigma can lead to discrimination. Nurses can also discriminate against patients based on stigma, e.g. discriminatory practices associated with people with HIV/AIDS or sexually transmitted infections. Being aware of the effects of discriminatory practices and striving to provide care that is fair and equitable can help the patient who may be feeling stigmatized.

Medications

There are certain medications (prescribed or recreational) which the patient may be taking that could have an effect on the individual's sexual potency and libido (Wakely 2001). Prescribed medications used to help with physical or psychological reactions to illness can cause sexual problems; such problems are termed 'iatrogenic'. Recreational drugs can lead to ejaculatory difficulties; a delay in orgasm and the desired loss of inhibition may lead to unsafe sex practices (Tomlinson 1999). When possible the nurse should advocate the use of safer sex activities and the use of condoms.

Most medications used for pain relief, e.g. codeine, can result in constipation. Feeling bloated and having a sense of fullness in the abdomen or rectum can impinge on sexuality. Constipation can cause weariness, lethargy and nausea, and may interfere with enjoyable vaginal and anal intercourse.

When assessing the patient's health needs, the nurse must be aware of the prescribed or non-prescribed medications that the patient is taking. The following lists some medications that may adversely affect the patient's sexual health (Gamlin 1999):

- Tobacco and alcohol
- Antihypertensives, e.g. propranolol and other β-adrenoreceptor blockers
- Certain diuretics, e.g. bendrofluazide and spironolactone
- H_2-receptor antagonists, e.g. cimetidine
- Proton pump inhibitors, e.g. omeprazole
- Anxiolytics, e.g. diazepam
- Antipsychotics, e.g. haloperidol
- Antiepileptics, e.g. carbamazepine.

Conclusions

Sexual health is central to each individual's well-being. Caring for patients in a holistic manner means that the nurse must also take into account the patient's sexual health needs. Nurses are often ideally placed to assess these. The art of effective communication, including the important aspect of listening, is paramount if care is to be truly holistic.

Sexuality is a very difficult concept to define and often nurses find it difficult to address the patient's sexual health needs. There may be several reasons for this, e.g. ignorance or embarrassment on the part of the nurse and/or the patient.

To help patients with problems related to sexual health, the nurse will need to obtain an in-depth sexual health history. For this to be done effectively and with confidence the nurse needs to develop her or his interpersonal and professional clinical skills. There are several barriers to effective sexual health care, e.g. perceived problems associated with the maintenance of confidentiality, embarrassment and lack of knowledge. Nurses need a skilled, unembarrassed and empathic approach in order to encourage patients to speak openly and freely about their problems. Patients may feel uneasy about asking questions because they may feel that they appear foolish or ignorant. As the nurse develops her or his repertoire of clinical nursing skills, asking intimate questions in a well-thought-out and caring manner will become easier and confidence will grow.

Disfiguring and mutilating surgery associated with the breasts, genitalia and reproductive organs, and traumatic events, e.g. a road traffic accident, can have a deleterious effect on the patient's self-esteem, self-image and sexuality. The outcome of such surgery or trauma (e.g. temporary or permanent changes) means that the nurse needs to deal with psychological and emotional issues. The nurse should encourage the patient to express fears and anxieties. The rehabilitative process is important in promoting adjustment and acceptance.

Finally, nurses need to know and understand that they do not have to be an expert on all problems with which patients may present. Many patients can be helped by the nurse being aware of her or his limitations and knowing where patients can be referred to outside the individual nurse's level of expertise.

References

Cairns, K.V. (1983) Sexual rehabilitation of gynaecological cancer patients. Sex Information and Education Council of Canada Newsletter 18(1).

Curtis, H., Hoolaghan, T. and Jewit, C. (1995) Sexual Health Promotion in General Practice. Oxford: Radcliffe.

de Marquiegui, A. and Huish, M. (1999) A woman's sexual life after an operation. In: Tomlinson, J. (ed.), The ABC of Sexual Health. London: BMJ Books, pp. 25–31.

Department of Health (2001) The National Strategy for Sexual Health and HIV: Maximising the opportunity. London: DoH.

Gamlin, R. (1999) Sexuality: A challenge for nursing practice. Nursing Times 95(7): 48–51.

Goffman, I. (1963) Stigma: Notes on the management of spoiled identity. Englewood Cliffs, NJ: Prentice-Hall.

Greenhouse, P. (1994) A sexual health service under one roof: setting up sexual health services for women. Journal of Maternal and Child Health 19: 228–233.

Ingram-Fogel, C. (1990) Human sexuality and health care: sexual health promotion. In: Ingram-Fogel, C. and Lauver, D. (eds), Sexual Health Promotion. Philadelphia: Saunders, pp. 1–38.

Jewitt, C. (1995) The HIV Project: Sexual history taking in general practice. London: The HIV Project.

Kinsey, A.C., Pomeroy, W.B., Martin, C.E. and Gebhard, P.H. (1948) Sexual Behaviour in the Human Male. Philadelphia: Saunders.

Kinsey, A.C., Pomeroy, W.B., Martin, C.E. and Gebhard, P.H. (1953) Sexual Behaviour in the Human Female. Philadelphia: Saunders.

Nursing and Midwifery Council (2002) Code of Professional Conduct. London: NMC.

Partridge, H. (1994) Changing faces: two years on. Nursing Standard 34(8): 54–58.

Peate, I. (1997) Taking a sexual health history: the role of the practice nurse. British Journal of Nursing 6: 978–983.

Riley, A. (1999) Sex in old age: continuing pleasure or continuing decline? Geriatric Medicine 29(3): 25–28.

Roberts, H. (2000) Sexuality expression for people with disfigurement. In: Wells, D. (ed.), Caring for Sexuality in Health and Illness. Edinburgh: Churchill Livingstone, pp. 226–239.

Rutter, M. (2000) The impact of illness on sexuality. In: Wells, D. (ed.), Caring for Sexuality in Health and Illness. Edinburgh: Churchill Livingstone, pp. 207–220.

Smeltzer, S.C. and Bare, B.G. (2000) Brunner and Suddarth's Textbook of Medical–Surgical Nursing, 9th edn. Philadelphia: Lippincott.

Tomlinson, J. (1999) Taking a sexual history. In: Tomlinson, J. (ed.), The ABC of Sexual Health. London: BMJ Books, pp. 12–15.

Wakely, G. (2001) Sexual problems in primary care. In: Carter, Y., Moss, C. and Weyman, A. (eds), Royal College of General Practitioners' Handbook of Sexual Health in Primary Care. London: RCGP, pp. 147–159.

Webb, C. (1985) Sexuality, Nursing and Health. Chichester: Wiley & Sons.

Weeks, J. (1993) Sexuality. London: Routledge.

Wells, D. (2000) Introduction. In: Wells, D. (ed.), Caring for Sexuality in Health and Illness. Edinburgh: Churchill Livingstone, pp. 1–7.

White, I. and Heath, H. (2002) Introduction. In: White, I. and Heath, H. (eds), The Challenge of Sexuality in Health Care. Oxford: Blackwell Science, pp. 3–11.

World Health Organization (1986) Concepts for Sexual Health. Copenhagen: WHO.

CHAPTER 14

Sleep and rest

DEBBIE DAVIES

Sleep is better than medicine.

English proverb

That we are not much sicker and much madder than we are is due exclusively to that most blessed and blessing of all natural graces – sleep.

Aldous Huxley (1950)

The capacity to rest and sleep is the right of every individual (Fox 1999). Quality sleep means that it is continuous and uninterrupted. As we get older sleep may be disrupted as a result of pain or discomfort, the need to go to the toilet, medical problems, medications, poorly organized work or social schedules, and sleep disorders (see www.sleepfoundation.org.uk). To nurse effectively, an awareness of the nature of sleep, and the factors that influence sleep and sleep problems, is essential in order to promote optimal sleep for the individual in a variety of care settings

What is sleep?

Sleep is a universal process common to all people. It is, according to Marieb (1995), 'a state of natural unconsciousness from which one can be aroused'. During this time, the processing of sensory input is minimal, coordinated behaviour eradicated, and cognitive activity such as thinking, planning and reflection suspended.

Sleep is a complicated physiological phenomenon that intrigues scientists. It takes up a significant component of the life span; about one-third of an individual's existence is spent in sleep. No human or animal has ever been shown to be able to go without sleep, although the amount needed varies.

Up until the 1950s sleep was considered to be a passive, dormant part of life associated with the simple withdrawal of wakefulness (National Institute of Neurological Disorders [NIND] 2003). More recently great strides have been made to clarify some of the mysteries of normal and abnormal sleep (Spangler 1997).

The use of the EEG (electroencephalogram) to measure brain activity revolutionized thinking about sleep, with the discovery of distinct sleep states where sleep is found to be a dynamic process during which the brain is very active (MacPherson 1994). Thus, there are recognized stages of sleep, each of which is characterized by a different type of brain activity.

As knowledge and information about physiological processes have developed, current views (Thompson et al. 2001) are that these distinct sleep states, actively generated by different brain regions, are now considered to exert significant and specific influences that affect most, if not all, fundamental homeostatic mechanisms.

Sleep, then, is not just a way of taking a respite from everyday busy routines; it is an essential component for good health, mental and emotional well-being, and personal safety (Jenson and Herr 1993). Indeed it has been clearly demonstrated that sleep loss or a sleep disorder can lead rapidly to impaired physiological function, deteriorating health and even death (Rechtschaffen et al. 1983), e.g. researchers have found that people with chronic sleep disorders are more likely to develop several types of psychiatric problems and to have higher blood pressure and suffer from excessive daytime sleepiness (Carskadon and Dement 1981, Wolfson and Carskadon 1998). Sleep loss influences the ability to undertake tasks that involve memory, learning and logical reasoning, leading to lost productivity, accidents, unsafe actions, strained relationships and unfulfilled potential.

Physiology of sleep

Sleep is controlled and regulated by two brain processes that respond to both internal and external stimuli (MacPherson 1994). The first is the restorative process when sleep occurs naturally in response to how long an individual is awake: the longer awake, the stronger the desire to sleep. The second process controls the timing of sleep and wakefulness during the day–night cycle and is known as the circadian rhythm or circadian biological clock.

Circadian rhythm

Circadian rhythms are regular changes in mental and physical characteristics that occur in the course of a day. Most circadian rhythms are controlled by the body's biological 'clock', a special centre in the hypothalamus of the brain known as the suprachiasmic nucleus (SCN).

Scientists have found that there is an association between staying awake during the day when it is light, and sleeping at night when it is dark (Fox 1999). Light that reaches photoreceptors in the retina of the eye creates signals that travel along the optic nerve to the SCN, which, by sending signals to several brain regions, in particular the pineal gland, works like a clock to set off activities affecting the whole body.

When exposed to the first light of day, the SCN initiates signals to these other parts of the brain associated with the sleep–wake cycle - hormone control, body temperature, urine production and blood pressure modification. Body temperature is raised, stimulating hormones such as cortisol. Blood levels of the hormone melatonin, which induces drowsiness and is associated with sleep onset, are much higher at night than in the day because production is suspended during daylight hours.

This 'clock' within the brain runs on a 24-hour cycle resulting in the feelings of sleepiness being at their strongest around 2.00–4.00am and in the afternoon between 1.00 and 3.00pm, thus influencing the timing and duration of sleep.

Circadian regularity begins by the third week of life. From the early months of wakefulness, during the early hours of the morning and late afternoon, by the time an infant is about 6 months old he or she will have developed a circadian rhythm that corresponds to the adult cycle.

When travellers pass from one time zone to another, they experience a disruption in the biological circadian rhythm that is known as 'jet lag', whereby the sufferer 'loses' time even though he or she may have slept. People who work shift patterns or nights will encounter similar symptoms.

The states and stages of sleep

Neurotransmitters and nerve-signalling chemicals control the sleep–wake cycle by acting on different groups of nerve cells, or neurons, in the brain. These will keep some parts of the brain active when the individual is awake. Others begin signalling as sleep begins, by 'switching off' those very signals.

As an individual sleeps, the sleep cycle passes through a range of differing, but predictable, states and stages throughout a typical 8-hour period. With continuous sleep each of these states alternates every 90 minutes.

Orthodox and paradoxical sleep

Orthodox sleep is described as sleep with non-rapid eye movement (NREM), which can be identified through four distinct progressive stages.

Paradoxical sleep is depicted as sleep with rapid eye movement (REM) and constitutes the fifth stage of the sleep cycle. Although the time spent in these states and stages will vary with age, it is generally agreed that 75% of the sleep cycle is NREM sleep and 25% REM sleep (Table 14.1).

For a restful and restorative sleep, the balance and mix of both REM and NREM are essential components of the sleep cycle, which takes up to 90–110 minutes to complete and occurs four to five times a night. As the night progresses, REM sleep periods increase in length whereas deep sleep decreases (Figure 14.1).

Table 14.1 Orthodox and paradoxical sleep

NREM sleep	As sleep commences, the stages of NREM or orthodox sleep progress. NREM sleep is considered to be essential for its restorative effects on the body
Stage 1	The eyes begin to close and the body relaxes. The eyes move very slowly and muscle activity is reduced. Sleep is light, drifting in and out, easily wakened. Mental activity is dream-like and if wakened many individuals remember fragmented visual images. There may also be the experience of sudden muscle contractions known as hypnic myoclonia, whereby there is often a sensation of falling before 'jumping' awake
Stage 2	Eye movements stop, with a slowing of brain activity. Breathing and heart rate become regular. Body temperature goes down. A person can still be easily roused
Stage 3	Delta sleep now occurs, whereby very slow brain waves begin to appear, intermingled with bursts of rapid waves known as sleep spindles. It is more difficult to wake someone in this stage
Stage 4	The deepest and most restorative sleep. Blood pressure drops, breathing slows and there is no eye movement or muscle activity. Energy is regained and hormones for growth and development are released. It is difficult to wake someone during this stage of sleep. If he or she is awakened the individual may spend some minutes feeling dazed and disoriented
REM sleep	The first REM sleep period takes place approximately 90 minutes after sleep has been initiated as the sleep pattern descends to a lower stage. During this time, vivid dreams occur, breathing and heart rate become more rapid and irregular, and there is transient limb immobility. The eyes periodically move rapidly from side to side. Males may develop penile erections. This stage of sleep is considered to be essential for effective daytime performance and may be associated with memory consolidation. Excessive lack of REM sleep is known to lead to hallucinations, paranoia and short-term personality changes

NREM, non-rapid eye movement; REM, rapid eye movement.

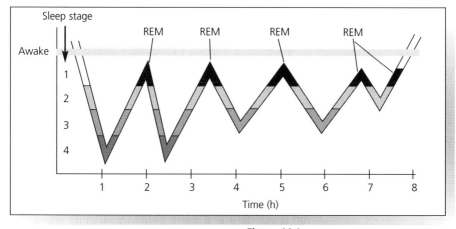

Figure 14.1
Stages of sleep.

Theories of the need for sleep

As more information and data are gathered by scientists in their quest to understand sleep, a number of theories are emerging to explain the function of sleep.

Developmental theory

Sleep plays a role in the development of the brain. REM sleep is a major component of sleep for babies *in utero* and infants. It has been suggested that, by activating visual, motor and sensory areas in the brain, sleep plays a role in preparing the individual for the outside world.

Conservation theory

It is physiologically vital to help the body recover from the work it does. By slowing down metabolism sleep enables the body to conserve and restore energy and may have some association with effective immune system function (Vitkovic et al. 2000). The physiological changes during NREM sleep include:

- arterial blood pressure falls
- pulse rate decreases
- peripheral blood vessels dilate
- skeletal muscle relaxes
- basal metabolic rate reduces.

Restorative theory

This theory hypothesizes that sleep can take place to enable physiological and biochemical repairs. According to this theory, sleep is necessary for the protein synthesis essential for cell growth and repair. This enables the central nervous system, more specifically neurons, to shut down and repair themselves. The secretion of growth hormone in children and young adults also occurs. Activity in parts of the brain associated with the control of emotions, decision-making processes and social interactions is also greatly reduced during deep sleep, which corresponds to optimal emotional and social functioning during waking hours.

Adaptive theory

This suggests that sleeping at night when vision is poor is a useful adaptive behaviour to protect individuals against predators.

Learning theories

During sleep, it is suggested that REM sleep plays a role in memory retention and consolidation. It also enables the brain to reorganize and store information.

The evidence suggests that, when deprived of REM sleep during a single night, retention of complex materials such as stories is greatly reduced. There are a number of proposed theories associated with the purpose of dreams and dreaming (Hobson 1998). These include: resolving emotional preoccupations, altering mood, in adaptation, in creativity and for amusement. One of the most long-standing notions, however, has been the link between dreaming and learning.

Dreaming and sleep

Modern scientific studies of the brain have led to discussion of a range of theories of sleep and its association with dreaming (Hobson and McCarley 1977, Crick and Mitchison 1983). It is estimated that an individual spends at least 2 hours each night dreaming. Dreaming takes place in a variety of ways, occurring at any stage during the four basic elements of the sleep cycle, although it occurs most commonly during periods of REM sleep, usually starting an hour and a half into sleep. It has been demonstrated that dreams are not always composed of just images. Blind people and people unable to visualize while awake also dream, their dreams being made up of mostly auditory and sensory experiences.

Originally, Sigmund Freud (1900), with his influence in the field of psychology, put forward the notion of dreaming as a 'safety valve' for unconscious worries and desires.

Some scientists consider dreams to be attempts by the cortex to find meaning in the random signals that it receives during REM sleep. By trying to interpret these signals a 'story' is created out of the fragmented brain activity (NIND 2003). Indeed Crick and Mitchison (1983) propose that dreams are the process of discarding unwanted memories, whereby information that is not required is wiped out by signals sent to the cortex. Winson (1990) suggests that dreaming enables the brain to process daily experiences into an ongoing strategy for behaviour, whereas others argue that dreaming gives the brain the opportunity to scan the environment in case of danger, incorporating the external stimuli into the dream.

There is general agreement, however, that for the most part dreaming is caused by internal biological processes. Which processes are responsible is open to debate. Of people who are wakened during REM sleep as many as 70–95% report dreams, in contrast to 5–10% of awakenings during NREM sleep. REM sleep is produced by the excretion of the chemical acetylcholine in the part of the brain stem known as the pons. Other neurotransmitters produced by the pons are able to switch off REM sleep. Conversely, there is evidence in some neurological literature that, in cases where there is loss of REM sleep, dreaming is still reported to occur, whereas, if there is damage to the frontal lobe of the brain, the REM cycle may be unaffected but dreaming is impossible. REM sleep is considered by some scientists to be only one of a number of dream triggers.

The study of lucid dreaming – the ability of the dreaming individual to become aware of the dream and be able to control it – is in its infancy and is one of the many challenges scientists face when exploring the mysteries of sleep and dreaming.

Sleep needs over the life cycle

Sleep needs vary. Sleep patterns are individual and may change but the need for sleep remains the same, a drive that must be met. Getting enough continuous uninterrupted quality sleep will contribute to short-term performance and feelings; it also impacts on the overall quality of our lives (Table 14.2).

Table 14.2 Sleep requirements and age

Infants/babies (includes naps)	0–2 months: 10.5–18.5 hours 2–12 months: 14–15 hours
Toddlers/children (includes naps)	12–18 months: 13–15 hours 18 months–3 years: 12–14 hours 3–5 years: 11–13 hours 5–12 years: 9–11 hours
Adolescents	8.5–9.5 hours
Adults/older people	On average: 7–9 hours

Although an average of 7–9 hours of sleep per night is generally recommended, the optimal amount will vary for each individual and over the life cycle. As can be seen in Table 14.2, newborns and infants require a lot of sleep and have several sleep periods throughout a 24-hour time cycle. This will include naps – which are important to children up to the age of 5 (see www.sleepfoundation.org.uk). As adolescence is reached, the sleep pattern shifts to a later sleep–wake cycle, with around 9 hours of sleep considered the optimum. Throughout adulthood and old age, patterns of sleep may change but 7–9 hours a night will ensure effective functioning (Figure 14.2).

Factors influencing sleep

According to Sorenson (1996), sleep disorders are common, serious, treatable and generally under-diagnosed. They cost the nation financially, have health and safety consequences, and cause decreased quality of life for many people. Sleep disorders can be categorized into primary sleep disorders, whereby the individual's sleep problem is the main disorder, and secondary sleep disorders. In this second situation the sleep problem is the

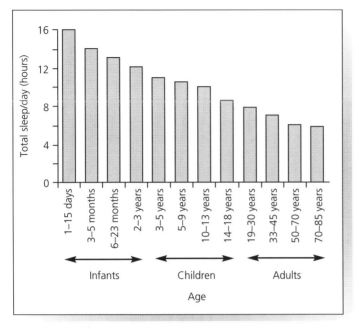

Figure 14.2 Ontogenetic development of the human sleep–dream cycle. (From Roffwarg et al. 1966.)

result of a distinct clinical disorder. All sleep and arousal disorders can be grouped into one of the following categories:

- Disorders of initiating and maintaining sleep
- Disorders of excessive somnolence
- Disorders of the sleep-wake schedule
- Dysfunctions associated with sleep, sleep stages or partial arousals.

An individual's ability to acquire the appropriate quality and quantity of sleep and to wake effectively is thus affected by a number of factors (Figure 14.3).

Psychological factors

Problems associated with sleep are considered to be closely related to mental health issues such as depression and schizophrenia. Anxiety and depression are often synonymous with sleep disturbance, of which early morning wakening is a significant feature. An individual with personal problems may be unable to relax sufficiently to get to sleep. Anxiety and excitement increase the production of noradrenaline (norepinephrine) blood levels, a chemical change that results in less stage 4 NREM sleep and REM sleep; there are more stage modifications and awakenings. In depressive conditions such as seasonal affective disorder (SAD) there may even be an increased quantity

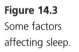

Figure 14.3
Some factors
affecting sleep.

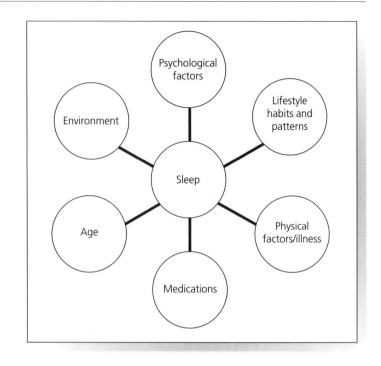

of sleep but of poor quality, which in turn increases fatigue. Post-traumatic stress disorder may lead to wakening by nightmares and an inability to return to sleep.

Sleep deprivation in itself can cause depression, even states of paranoia and hallucinations. It may also influence the symptoms of mental disorder, e.g. episodes of agitation in people with manic depression.

Motivation, the desire to stay awake, may often overcome a person's fatigue and even if tired the individual will stay awake if something interesting is going on. By contrast, without the motivation to stay awake, a person who is bored is more likely to fall asleep.

Lifestyle habits and patterns

Situations that disrupt circadian rhythms will influence the quality and quantity of sleep that an individual achieves. A person who does shift work and changes shifts frequently may experience sleep disturbances.

Many blind people have sleep disorders because they cannot detect light and so their biological clock does not follow the normal 24-hour light-induced clock. Jet lag is also a common cause of sleep disruption. Moderate exercise is considered to be conducive to sleep but excessive exercise may stimulate the sympathetic nervous system, resulting in difficulty in getting to sleep.

The use of chemicals/substances will influence sleep and the sleep cycle. Beverages that contain caffeine, such as coffee, tea and fizzy drinks, act as stimulants of the nervous system and thus disrupt sleep. Although initially hastening the onset of sleep, excessive alcohol intake actually disrupts REM sleep, creating a rebound effect when the individual either wakes when the effects of alcohol wear off or has vivid dreams or nightmares. Nicotine also has a stimulant effect on the nervous system. Many smokers describe themselves as light sleepers.

Bedtime rituals and routines influence an individual's ability to sleep effectively – good sleep hygiene routines assist the individual to have a good night's sleep, by creating a period of calmness and relaxation; this may include the time of going to bed and a warm bath before bedtime. Reduction in stimulating situations will also encourage a good sleep routine. Going to bed when moderately tired is likely to lead to a restful sleep rather than when being overtired.

A warm milky drink, which contains dietary L-trytophan, an amino acid thought to induce sleep, is often used to promote sleepiness, as do peanut butter, cheese and nuts.

Environmental factors

The environment in which the individual seeks to sleep and rest is an important consideration. A familiar bedroom, bed, pillows, type of bed-clothes, degree of light/dark, for example, will influence how well an individual sleeps.

Changes to the environment such as excessive, sharp or intermittent strange sounds and noise, extremes of heat and cold, a poorly ventilated room, unfamiliar surroundings, and the issues associated with hospitalization are examples of factors that may disrupt sleep. Continuous care, treatment schedules and hospital routines lend credence to the old adage about patients being roused from sleep by the nurse in order to take a sleeping tablet! Sleeping with or without someone may influence sleep patterns – many people have slept together in the same bed for a number of years; others may find that a clinical environment where there is a group of strangers is stressful. Indeed the relevance of the environment to sleep within the clinical context was explored in depth by Florence Nightingale as long ago as 1860 (Nightingale 1860).

Physical factors and the lifespan

As has been demonstrated, there are developmental sleep requirements associated with age. Although the amount of sleep required will vary between individuals there are some general considerations that can be applied; life cycle changes are likely to influence sleep. Pregnant women are likely to need more sleep, particularly during the first 3 months of pregnancy.

Having a new baby or small children will affect the ability to attain an undisturbed night's rest.

Getting too little sleep over a period of time creates a 'sleep debt' – even if an individual gets used to a sleep-depriving way of life, judgement and reaction time continue to be disrupted.

Changes in the life cycle, such as menopause, exhibit symptoms such as insomnia. There is a tendency for people who are older to sleep more lightly and for a shorter time span, although it is generally agreed that they need the same amount of sleep as when they were in early adulthood. There is evidence that about half of all people over the age of 65 have sleeping problems such as insomnia and the deep sleep stages essential to sleep often become reduced or stop completely. This change may be considered to be a normal part of ageing or result from medical problems associated with age, bladder problems and lack of mobility.

Illness and disease

Illness and disease can have an effect on sleep and sleep-related disorders. The converse can also occur when the process of sleep may itself influence the disease/illness process. In these situations sleep onset may be prevented and wakefulness may occur, or there may be difficulties with positioning or the need to eliminate.

During illness the individual often requires more sleep. Neurons that control sleep interact with the immune system. Potent sleep-inducing chemicals, known as cytokines, are produced by the immune system at the onset of infections such as influenza. These may enable the body to conserve energy and use its resources to fight the illness.

The pain, discomfort and fatigue caused by illness or medical intervention such as surgery may adversely affect sleep by either preventing sleep or wakening the sleeper. The impact of illness on an individual can create fear and anxiety, disrupt day/night routines, and in its wider context impact adversely on caregivers too.

The scope of medical problems that influence sleep and sleep patterns is wide ranging. The exacerbation of asthma, for example, or the onset of an acute cerebrovascular accident, has a propensity to occur more frequently at night, possibly as a result of the physiological changes associated with sleep that have previously been identified (see www.ninds.nih.gov/health).

Some types of epilepsy are also affected by sleep. Sleep deprivation may trigger a seizure, on the one hand, but another form of epileptic seizure may be exacerbated by deep sleep. REM sleep appears to help contain the spread of a seizure that originates in a confined region of the brain. Patients with neurological conditions such as Alzheimer's disease and head injury are also likely to experience problems with sleeping. This may be caused by changes in regions of the brain and neurotransmitters that control sleep or by drugs used to control symptoms of the disorder.

Breathing difficulties such as shortness of breath, nasal congestion, a cough associated with acute and/or chronic respiratory conditions, and cardiac disorders such as congestive cardiac failure are likely to lead to sleep disturbance (Closs 1989). This in turn leads to an increase in fatigue that perpetuates the cycle of distress. Up to 45% of cancer patients have serious sleep disturbances (Katz and McHarney 1998). Gastrointestinal problems such as reflux or peptic ulcers cause pain and discomfort, often as the result of an increase in gastric secretions associated with REM sleep.

Medications

There are a number of groups of medications that influence the sleep-wake cycle. Examples of these include: hypnotics, which can interfere with the latter stages of sleep and REM sleep, and affect the quality of sleep; some drugs used in cardiology, e.g. β blockers, are known to cause vivid dreams, nightmares and insomnia; many drugs interfere with or suppress REM sleep – morphine, a narcotic, causes frequent awakenings and drowsiness, and tranquillizers, amphetamines and antidepressants may also exhibit these properties.

Medications given to help patients sleep act by either inducing sleep or reducing anxiety. One of the side effects of these drugs is an increased tolerance and over-reliance, which may lead people to increase the drug dose or supplement it with alcohol. Other side effects are often exacerbated in elderly clients as a result of their altered rates of metabolism, absorption and body fat (Kozier et al. 1998). As a consequence, there has been a shift towards alternative ways of promoting sleep without the use, or with only limited use, of medication.

Common primary sleep disorders

Among the more common sleep disorders are insomnia, sleep apnoea, narcolepsy, restless legs syndrome and the parasomnias.

Insomnia

The most common sleep disorder is insomnia, whereby people complain of inadequate or poor quality sleep because of one or more of the following (Doghrami 1999):

- Falling asleep with difficulty
- Waking frequently during the night with difficulty returning to sleep
- Premature waking
- Not feeling refreshed on waking.

Insomnia can be classified as transient if it lasts for only up to a couple of weeks, and intermittent if transient insomnia occurs from time to time (Katz and McHarney 1998). In these situations the sleep disorder is often associated with the influencing factors outlined previously. Insomnia is chronic if it occurs on most nights and lasts a month or more, when the actual cause of the sleep changes may have been resolved.

The condition affects both men and women but is the most common sleep-related complaint for women (Doghrami 1999). It often disrupts the individual's daily life. When it occurs, tiredness is a key issue and there is a tendency to worry about not getting enough sleep.

The use of sleep medication is deemed questionable when seeking to resolve insomnia, particularly in the long term when it is argued that the situation can be made worse (Long et al. 1993; see www.ninds.nih.gov).

Treatment for insomnia therefore has its focus on the development of new behavioural patterns to reduce sleep disturbance. It may take several months to reset the sleep–wake cycle using a plan that may have a range of interchangeable elements related to daytime activities, preparation for sleep and interpretation of the sleep experience.

Sleep apnoea

Sleep apnoea, from the Greek word for 'want of breath', is a disorder of interrupted breathing during sleep, where airflow at the nose and mouth is absent for 10 seconds to a minute while the sleeping individual struggles to breathe.

The condition can be classified as obstructive, central or mixed, depending on the presence or absence of respiratory muscle effort. People with apnoea are deprived of oxygen during sleep, although the severity of the decrease in oxygen saturation will vary (Khawaja and Phillips 1998).

In obstructive apnoea, airflow is physically blocked but abdominal and ribcage efforts continue. It usually occurs in conjunction with fat build-up or loss of muscle tone associated with ageing, and is common in men. There may also be airway problems such as enlarged tonsils or jaw abnormalities. In central apnoea, which is thought to be neurological rather than physical in origin and which is more common in women, both types of movement are absent.

During an episode of obstructive apnoea, efforts to inhale air create a suction that then causes collapse of the windpipe. These involuntary cycles may be as high as 20–30 per hour throughout the night, usually associated with loud snoring in between apnoeic episodes, as the blood oxygen levels fall; the brain responds by waking up the individual enough to tighten the upper airway muscles and open the trachea. The person may snort or gasp and then continue to snore, although not everyone who snores has sleep apnoea.

As a consequence, many people with sleep apnoea describe it as a choking sensation which, with the frequent awakenings, leads to complaints of morning headaches, daytime sleepiness, irritability or depression, and loss of libido (Khawaja and Phillips 1998). At its most serious, sleep apnoea is linked to high blood pressure, irregular heartbeats, increased risk of cardiovascular catastrophe and even respiratory arrest.

Treatments vary following diagnosis and range from weight loss, encouraging the individual to sleep on their side, and advice not to use alcohol, tobacco or sleep medication. More complex treatments may involve the use of devices such as nasal continuous positive airway pressure (CPAP), dental appliances or surgery to correct the obstruction.

Narcolepsy

Narcolepsy is a chronic sleep disorder that may be genetic in origin; the main characteristic is excessive and overwhelmingly irresistible daytime sleepiness, even with a normal amount of night-time sleep. Symptoms usually appear during adolescence (see www.ninds.nih.gov).

A less common symptom of narcolepsy is cataplexy, an abrupt reversible loss of muscle function brought on by strong emotions such as fright, laughter or anger. The individual remains conscious throughout.

Sleep paralysis, also associated with narcolepsy, is a terrifying experience that occurs just before waking up or falling asleep, where there is a temporary inability to talk or move. Often accompanied by vivid frightening hypnagogic hallucinations, sleep paralysis terminates spontaneously after a few minutes.

The most effective treatment is with drug therapy such as central nervous system stimulants or tricyclic antidepressants. Daytime naps may help with daytime alertness.

Restless legs syndrome

A common, familial disorder found particularly among elderly people, and pregnant and premenopausal women, which involves unpleasant sensations in the legs and feet, variously described as creeping, crawling, tingling or pulling. Although not described as painful, the urge to move the limb is overwhelming. Restless legs syndrome (RLS) can be experienced when awake or asleep and not necessarily in bed, but is associated with insomnia. Many of those with this disorder also experience a related sleep disorder called periodic limb movements in sleep (PLMS), in which involuntary jerking of the limbs at frequent intervals leads to difficulties with falling asleep and with maintaining sleep, leading to daytime sleepiness.

Parasomnias

Parasomnias refers to the group of arousal behaviours that may interfere with sleep. Examples of a range of these dysfunctions are:

- Nocturnal enuresis (bedwetting during sleep) is often associated with children aged over 3 years, occurring 1-2 hours after falling asleep, when moving from stage 3 to 4 of NREM sleep. It is more common in males.

- Somnambulism (sleepwalking) occurs during stages 3 and 4 of NREM sleep 1–2 hours after falling asleep. Episodic sleepwalkers require protection from danger.
- Sleep talking occurs during NREM sleep just before REM sleep.
- Nocturnal erections and emissions occur during REM sleep, starting in adolescence.
- Bruxism – clenching and grinding of teeth – usually occurs during stage 2 NREM sleep.

Promoting sleep

With the concept of individualized patient care as the cornerstone of modern professional nursing in society (Roper et al. 1990), the interrelationship of sleep, health and the patient experience should be of great relevance when undertaking holistic care. As Jenson and Herr (1993) point out, the role of the nurse is essential in the thorough assessment of sleep patterns, the identification of requirements and the implementation of effective activities to enhance healthy sleep.

Good communication skills, the use of formal assessment tools to identify needs and problems, and an individualized care programme, which when implemented and evaluated ensure optimal sleep as an essential component of health and well-being, are key to effective nursing.

Nursing assessment

The initial nursing assessment may take the form of obtaining a complete sleep history from the client. Initially the history may be part of the general information gathered in order to plan care to specific needs and preferences. A more detailed history would be required if there is an indication that there is a sleep problem. This would establish the exact nature of the problem, its effect on the client, and the success or otherwise of strategies in use to overcome it. General information elicited will include the following:

- Usual sleeping pattern
- Bedtime rituals
- Use of sleep medication
- Effective sleep environment
- Recent changes in sleep pattern.

If there has been a change in pattern or difficulty with sleeping, a more detailed history that explores the nature of the problem should be ascertained. This may include questions that:

- clarify what happens at sleep onset
- determine the extent of excessive daytime sleepiness

- characterize the extent and content of awakenings
- delineate sleep habits
- review intake of chemical substances such as alcohol
- establish the possibility of obstructive sleep apnoea.

Other nursing assessment tools may be brought into play, e.g. the keeping of a sleep diary to obtain more detailed and precise information about a particular problem. There is a range of scales that can be used to gain objective data for assessment, e.g. the Epworth Sleepiness Scale (1991) and the Stansford Sleepiness Scale (Hoddes et al. 1972).

A physical examination by the nurse will elicit information to determine the extent of the problem. Examples are whether the client looks fatigued, lacks energy, has darkened rings or puffiness around the eyes, is exhibiting irritable behaviours or confusion, or has a deviated nasal septum.

Planning care

The major outcome for the client will be the maintenance or re-establishment of a sleep pattern that enables the client to wake refreshed and able to have enough energy to complete day-to-day activities. The range of nursing strategies and interventions identified will reflect an understanding of the client's individual situation or problem.

Implementing care

Assisting the client to sleep, particularly in the formal hospital setting, requires the nurse to be creative with knowledge and understanding about the nature of sleep and its relevance to the individual. The following are key interventions to explore:

- The creation of a restful environment by reducing environmental distractions. Ensuring that the client feels physically and psychologically safe within the environment.
- Supporting accustomed bedtime rituals.
- Promoting comfort and relaxation.
- Administering appropriate sleep medication.
- Client teaching – new strategies to aid sleep, e.g. relaxation techniques.

Evaluation

Success of client outcomes should be established through observation, monitoring and questioning. Observation of the duration of sleep, signs of NREM and REM sleep, and elicitation of the client's feelings about how they feel, and the success or failure of specific strategies, are key to evaluation.

Conclusion

Although the notion of sleep and rest is often one of the last activities of living to be considered, it is certainly not inconsequential. It has been clearly established that sleep is a complex phenomenon, the functions of which are essential to health, well-being and even survival. A knowledge and understanding about the nature of sleep and the factors associated with sleep and sleep problems should be part of every nurse's repertoire. This will enable the nurse to consider objectively and creatively successful strategies to promote optimal sleep for each individual.

References

Carskadon, M.A. and Dement, W.C. (1981) Cumulative effects of sleep restriction on daytime sleepiness. Psychophysiology 18: 107–113.

Closs, J. (1989) Patients' sleep–wake rhythms in hospital. Parts 1 and 2. Nursing 84: 48–50, 54–55.

Crick, F. and Mitchison, G. (1983) The function of dream sleep. Nature 304: 111–114.

Doghrami, K. (1999) Clinical frontiers in the sleep/psychiatry interface. Psychiatry Treatment Updates Medscape Inc. Satellite Symposium in American Psychiatric Association Meeting, 22 June, pp. 1–13.

Epworth Sleepiness Scale (1991) Measurement of sleep deprivation. Sleep 14: 540–545.

Fox, M. (1999) The importance of sleep. Nursing Standard 13(24): 44–47.

Freud, S. (1900) The Interpretations of Dreams. Cited in Brill, E.J. (ed., trans.) (1938) The Basic Writings of Sigmund Freud. New York: Modern Library, pp. 251–252.

Hobson, J. (1998) The Dreaming Brain. New York: Basic Books.

Hobson, J. and McCarley, R.W. (1977) The brain as a dream state generator. American Journal of Psychiatry 134: 1335–1368.

Hoddes, E., Deent, W. and Zarcone, V. (1972) The development and use of the Stanford Sleepiness Scale. Psychophysiology 9: 150.

Huxley, A. (1950) Variations on a philosopher. In: Huxley, A., Themes and Variations. New York: Harper & Brothers.

Jenson, D.P. and Herr, K.A. (1993) Sleeplessness: advances in clinical nursing research. Nursing Clinics of North America 26: 385–405.

Katz, D. and McHarney, C. (1998) Clinical correlates of insomnia in patients with chronic illness. Archives of Internal Medicine 158: 1099–1107.

Khawaja, I. and Phillips, B. (1998) Obstructive sleep apnoea: diagnosis and treatment. Hospital Medicine 34(3): 33–36, 39–41.

Kozier, B., Erb, G., Blais, K. and Wilkinson, J. (1998) Rest and sleep. In: Fundamentals of Nursing: Concepts, process and practice, 5th edn. Redwood City, CA: Addison Wesley Longman Inc., pp. 952–969.

Long, B., Phipps, W. and Cassmeyer, V. (1993) Sleep disorders. In: Medical–Surgical Nursing. A Nursing Process Approach. St Louis, MI: Year Book.

MacPherson, G. (ed.) (1994) Black's Medical Dictionary, 37th edn. London: A&C Black.

Marieb, E. (1995) Essentials of Human Anatomy and Physiology, 3rd edn. London: Mosby.

National Institute of Neurological Disorders (2003) National Institutes of Health: US Department of Health and Human Services (www.ninds.nih.gov/health/sleepbasics).

Nightingale, F. (1860) Notes on nursing. What it is and what it is not. In: Ockerbloom, M.M. (ed.), A Celebration of Women Writers (www.celebration@pobox.upennedu).

Rechtschaffen, A., Gilliland, M., Bergmann, B. and Winter, J. (1983) Physiological correlates of prolonged sleep deprivation in rats. Science 221: 182–184.

Roffwarg, H.P. et al. (1966) Ontogenetic development of the human sleep–dream cycle. Science 152: 604–619.

Roper, N., Logan, W. and Tierney, A. (1990) The Elements of Nursing: A model of living, 3rd edn. Edinburgh: Churchill Livingstone.

Sorenson, D.S. (1996) Sleep module: http://learn.sdstate.edu/sorensond/nurs760Fall02

Spangler, F.A. (1997) The Neurobiology of Sleep. Cambridge: Cambridge Scientific Abstracts.

Thompson, S., Ackerman, U. and Horner, R. (2001) Sleep as a teaching tool for integrating respiratory physiology and motor control. Advances in Physiological Education 25: 29–44.

Vitkovic, L. et al. (2000) Inflammatory cytokines. Journal of Neurochemistry 74: 457–471.

Winson, J. (1990) The meaning of dreams. Scientific American 262: 86–89.

Wolfson, A.R. and Carskadon, M.A. (1998) Sleep schedules and daytime functioning in adolescents. Child Development 69: 875–887.

Websites

www.apsa.org/pubinfo/remaque.htm (accessed 19/07/04)

www.macalesteredu.org (accessed 16/07/04)

www.ninds.nih.gov/health/sleepbasics (accessed 30/06/04)

www.sleepfoundation.org (accessed 30/06/04)

CHAPTER 15
Death and dying

MARY GREENO

This chapter considers the care of a person facing death and loss. The psychological, physical, spiritual and religious needs, and social support are addressed. The term 'patient' is used throughout this chapter because it sets the relationship between the carer and the person for whom he or she cares.

There are different types of death. There is the expected death that may be caused by a terminal illness or old age, or a sudden or unexpected death that may result from a car accident or a sudden acute illness, such as a heart attack or stroke.

Although we may become familiar with death and caring for the dying patient, the nurse must remember that for the patient and his or her family it is a singularly unique experience. This experience may be painful, unfamiliar and frightening.

When a patient is dying it is important that her or his self-esteem be preserved and personal dignity not violated. She or he must feel in control of her or his own destiny. Some of the nursing care that we provide may undermine her or his modesty and personal privacy; however, this can be minimized by explaining the procedure to be undertaken, so that there is understanding and cooperation through obtaining informed consent. For example, if the patient needs an enema to relieve constipation, this procedure, similar to catheterization, can be very embarrassing for the patient. To minimize embarrassment, expose the minimum amount of the patient's body and make sure that the curtain or door is closed, to ensure patient privacy.

Caring for a dying patient can take place at home, in a hospital or in a hospice. Wherever it occurs, there should be adequate support systems in place for patients, relatives and staff. Where possible this can be achieved through a multidisciplinary approach. It must be remembered that the relationships staff form in order to care for patients will cause some form of sadness or grief for them when death finally occurs.

By using examples of how people avoid talking about death, Freud (1918) claimed that no person really believed in his or her own mortality, clarifying that 'the aim of all life is death'. Jung (1959) stressed the value of beliefs about death and their importance for daily life. He claimed that the first part of one's life is concerned with the preparation for the life ahead and the second half with the preparation for death. Nursing is at the forefront of matters concerned with dying and death, and nurses are expected to become competent when caring.

Where to die

Most people wish to die at home if there is appropriate help available. If people live alone then home care may include:

- family support
- district/community nurses
- night sitters
- specialist nurses such as the Macmillan nurses
- general practitioners
- respite care.

The district/community nurse's success at arranging maximum home support from all agencies is vital. He or she also needs expertise in symptom control if hospital admissions are to be avoided.

Hospital may be a secure place for some people who have had recurrent treatments. Hospice-attached day centres offer special treatments and social support for those living alone and for all patients and their families. However, the ability to return home nightly helps the patient to maintain independence for as long as possible. Hospice care is a philosophy of care that should spread throughout every hospital and primary care team. Admissions are frequently for symptom control or family respite.

Some of the losses a dying patient or the family may experience

Patients may experience loss of health, weight, mobility, independence, financial income, youth, dignity, and a role within the family and community. The family may experience the loss of a family member, home, financial income, security and company.

The death of a loved one brings with it the greatest experience of loss. Grief is frequently described as a feeling of deep sorrow associated with this loss. Grieving is described as the state of feeling grief, and bereavement is described as the time span during which this occurs.

It is commonly recognized that the person left behind is the one experiencing grief but it must be recognized that, when patients are facing their own death, they may experience many losses: the loss of their own life, leaving their loved ones behind, the hopes, dreams and expectations that may be unfulfilled.

If the relatives know in advance that their loved one is going to die, they may start their grieving before the death occurs in anticipation of the event. It is good if both the patient and the family can support each other by exploring the grieving path together. This can be achieved through openness, and not secrecy.

The nurse's role at this time is to support both the patient and the family through the pain and grief. People may show their pain in many ways.

Family involvement

Some families do not want anyone else involved in the care of the dying person but themselves, because they may fear that the nurse will not be gentle enough with their loved one and may try to take over the caring role. Many families may want to do the nursing and only want to be shown how to move the patient and carry out pressure care.

Nurses must respect the families' commitment and never take over. Their role is to teach, encourage and support the family, carry out the nursing care, reassuring them that they are doing the right thing. In this way, nurses can lessen regrets rather than increase them. A peaceful death can be a lasting comfort to the family.

There are many theoretical approaches relating to the dying process. Kubler-Ross (1969) classified the 'stages model'. She identified five stages that dying people were understood to go through. The stages of dying are a pattern of thinking and behaving that most people go through after learning they are dying. Kubler-Ross (1969) states that not all patients react the same or move through the stages in the same way or at the same time.

Denial

This is the first stage, when the patient is first diagnosed and told that the illness will lead to death, and which he or she may refuse to believe. It is a temporary defence against the overwhelming news. There may be a 'grasping at straws'. Sometimes reality can be faced but often not for long and not too frequently. Acceptance has to be in the heart as well as in the head.

Anger

In the second stage, the patient feels angry and resentful. It is marked by the phrase: 'It's not fair, why me?' This anger can be directed at anyone: God, hospitals, nurses or doctors. This can be a difficult stage for the family, friends and carers. There can be periods of fear and agitation, and support should be given to the patient during these times.

Bargaining

This has been identified as the third stage; the patient is calmer but attempts to bargain with God or a supreme being, making promises if death will be postponed.

Depression or anticipatory grief

This is the fourth phase. Kubler-Ross (1969) claims that the patient starts to accept dying and feels sadness and grief, and may start mourning for the imminent loss of life.

Acceptance

During this stage the patient has accepted the inevitability of death and may feel peaceful about it or may become withdrawn. The acceptance of death by both patient and family is a painful pathway that can be trodden only a little at a time. Some people pass silently along the pathway, coming to terms with death inside themselves, voicing little of their thoughts, whereas others voice their feelings and reactions. However, for some it is not a happy state, but an end to the struggle.

It is important to remember that the dying person need not go through all the phases and not necessarily in the order outlined above. According to Thompson (2002), this model has come in for considerable criticism. He identified that it has much in common with work developed later by Murray-Parkes (1986), who also favoured a stages approach – discussed later.

The needs of the dying patient

Dying patients appear to share some common fears:

• pain and suffering
• loneliness and dying alone
• fear for their relatives and how they will cope
• fear about what happens after death.

When nursing terminally ill patients, the nurse must remember that the emphasis moves from curative to palliative care.

Palliative care must include up-to-date knowledge of the therapy required to achieve good symptom control. It is unacceptable that anyone should suffer severe pain or distress during a final illness. The nurse's role is to ensure that he or she has the skills and knowledge required to achieve this goal, otherwise the symptom control team in a hospital or the hospice team in the community can be requested to advise.

Models of bereavement began to emerge from the late 1960s onwards in the work of authors such as Kubler-Ross (1969) and Murray-Parkes (1986). Their work, according to Hockey (1990), was a result of articles written and published by Dame Cicely Saunders on the care of dying people.

Murray-Parkes (1986) identifies the five stages of grief as: (1) alarm, (2) searching, (3) anger/guilt, (4) despair and (5) gaining a new identity.

A dying patient may experience feelings of isolation for various reasons. Fears are expressed about dying by suffocating or choking and some patients are afraid to sleep for fear of failing to wake up. Patients may feel unable to share their thoughts about dying and are left alone with their emotions and fears. Buckman (2000) says that, once patients have begun to speak their thoughts, feelings and fears, it is important to let them do so at their own pace. Reflecting back on their statements, ensuring correct interpretation of what they are conveying, shows that you are actually listening. The use of non-verbal cues, e.g. nodding, encourages them to continue. At this time it is important that the patient and family talk to each other (if this is what they wish), so that their affairs may be put in order, because unfinished business may cause distress for both patients and their families.

Beauchamp and Childress (2001) identified four ethical principles that must be adhered to by all nurses; these are: (1) autonomy, (2) beneficence, (3) non-maleficence and (4) justice.

When considering patient autonomy, it is the patient's right to make decisions about his or her care. Patients should always be involved in planning their care and it is their right to accept or refuse any nursing or medical intervention. Beneficence is to do good or provide benefits to others, whereas non-maleficence dictates that we do no harm to others. Justice means that everyone receives a fair share of the available resources, namely they should receive care according to their needs.

Bradbury (2000) claims that western society sees a good death as one where the patient does not suffer. This should be the aim of every nurse, to ensure that the patient is pain free and comfortable. The nurse should ensure that patients' physical, psychological, cultural and religious beliefs are respected and their individual needs met. It is important that patients are given time to discuss any fears about their imminent death. All questions should be answered truthfully with sensitivity and maintenance of patient confidentiality at all times to ensure trust.

Caring for patients who are dying and their relatives can be an alarming prospect, but for some nurses it is one of the most rewarding and fulfilling aspects of nursing practice. Often, it is envisaged that the people you care for will get better; however, Henderson (1996) says the nurse's unique position is to assist individuals, sick or well, in the performance of their activities, contributing to health or recovery or to a peaceful death.

It must be remembered that every person is a unique individual, with his or her own personality, social, cultural and spiritual background and life experiences. The nurse must address the needs of the whole person through providing holistic care – body, mind and soul in unison.

Family members should be supported if they wish to participate in caring for their loved ones. They may wish to assist in bathing the patient, administering mouth care, giving sips of water or feeding the patient. Adams (1997) says, however, that control of the patient's symptoms becomes the main issue whether the patient is cared for at home, in a hospice or in hospital. Accurate assessment of the patient's needs is essential for good symptom control, which does not refer just to pain control; as Dickenson et al. (2000) point out, there may also be emotional pain and other symptoms such as nausea, constipation and breathlessness.

Wilson (2004) states that terminally ill patients would prefer to die at home, or to spend as much time there as possible. For the dying person and the family, this can be a rewarding experience; however, it can also be both physically and emotionally draining. The community nursing services, the Macmillan nurse or the Marie Curie nurse can be accessed for support and respite so that the family can get some rest.

Hockey (1990) claims that generally death in old age is a prolonged gradual process from a multitude of ailments rather than one exact disease. MacDonald describes her experience of being 70 years old in MacDonald and Rich (1984):

> One does not just die all of a sudden. It is a process and one we may be conscious of for the last ten or twenty years of our life which, if you think about it, may be a quarter or more of your lifetime. I find myself wondering why this is not more talked about and why it has not become the common knowledge of our lives. I am self-conscious in writing this, for after all no one speaks of dying until they have only a few months or weeks or hours to live. This is society's definition of dying. It asks that I deceive myself and others about my daily awareness that my body is using itself up; prevents me from calling this process by name for myself and others.

MacDonald identifies the fact that many aspects of ageing are hidden in western society because together the physical and mental concomitants are not socially accepted.

Some dying patients may fear being isolated both physically and psychologically. Some do not like being in a room alone; they prefer to be surrounded by people and the general activity of the ward. However, mental isolation can be very painful, if the patient is afraid to discuss impending death with his or her family or carers for fear of breaking down. The patient should be encouraged by the nurse to talk. The nurse should be relaxed and unhurried when carrying out any procedure; good communication skills are essential in every aspect of nursing, but more so when caring for the dying patient and his or her family.

Good practice in caring for patients and relatives/friends before death

- Always welcome the relatives, irrespective of the time of day or night
- Respect and value their participation in caring for their loved one
- Respect patients' needs, having regard for their spiritual beliefs and culture
- All nursing care must be based on patients' individual needs.

If the family is with the patient 24 hours a day, a single room may be appropriate to ensure privacy. However, if the patient does not have anyone sitting with him or her, then the main ward may be appropriate so that the patient is never alone and someone sits with him or her during the last hours of his or her life.

The aim in the care of the dying patient is to provide care that relieves the patient of pain, so that death comes in a gentle way and with dignity. This can be achieved only if the needs of the body, mind and soul are met together. The nurse must always remember that patients' attitudes towards death vary a great deal. Cultural and religious beliefs will influence this and the spiritual needs of the patient should be respected and addressed. The nurse must remember that practices vary within each religion and culture; the nurse should always consult the patient or family about religious observances to ensure that no offence is inadvertently caused. Death may come quickly or slowly depending on the patient and his or her condition. The nurse must continue to provide care up to and after death.

Buckman, in Dickenson et al. (2000), identified some of the fears experienced by staff when caring for terminally ill patients and their relatives:

- Fear of causing pain
- Fear of being blamed
- Fear of not knowing the answers
- Fear of unleashing and having to respond to strong reactions
- Fear of expressing personal feelings
- Fear of having to confront own fears of illness and mortality
- Fear of reaction from peers (who may not always be supportive).

Signs of approaching death

- The patient may feel cold regardless of the room temperature and the number of blankets covering him or her.
- The patient may seem to become peaceful, not showing any signs of discomfort.
- Consciousness may give way to semi-consciousness/unconsciousness, with the patient drifting in and out of consciousness until eventually drifting into a coma. However, some patients may be conscious until death.
- The nurse must always remember that the sense of hearing is the last sense to be lost, so the room where the patient is being cared for, or the area of the ward, should be quiet.
- The patient's circulation may slow down, making the patient's skin appear pale and possibly cold to touch.
- The patient's pulse may become weak and irregular and you may be unable to feel it before the patient dies.
- The patient's breathing may become irregular and laboured and the patient may develop Cheyne–Stokes breathing, where big gaps between breaths occur until the patient stops breathing altogether. Mucus in the throat and airways may make a sound that is often called 'a death rattle'.

- In some patients the muscles may relax and the patient's body becomes limp.
- There is no pulse, respiration or blood pressure.
- The pupils are fixed and dilated.

Procedures after death

The following procedures may be undertaken after the death of the patient:

- The doctor or general practitioner in the community must be called to certify that the patient is dead.
- Confirmation of death must be recorded in both the medical and the nursing notes.
- Depending on the ward's protocol, the nurse may proceed gently to lay the patient flat on the bed with one pillow.
- Dentures must be inserted into the mouth immediately because it may be difficult later when rigor mortis sets in.
- The patient's eyes are closed.
- A pillow or a rolled-up towel is placed on the patient's chest under the chin to support the jaw.
- The patient's arms and legs are straightened.
- Remove any mechanical aids such as syringe drivers unless otherwise stated, e.g. in the case of an unexpected death that will be referred to the coroner.
- The body is covered with a clean sheet and left for an hour, or whatever the ward's protocol is, before the last offices are performed. The last offices are when the body is prepared for removal to the mortuary.

If the relatives are not present at the time of death, the nurse must have ascertained previously if they wished to be called any time of the day or night when the event happens. Thayre and Peate (2003) claim that when contacting and notifying relatives of the death of their loved one the first step in breaking bad news is very important. They claim that it may present a dilemma as to whether you tell them over the telephone in order to avoid a distressed dash to the hospital, or by saying that the condition of their loved one had deteriorated and could they come to the hospital where the news of the death can be broken in a more gentle way. Thayre and Peate (2003) provide suggestions for a nurse's first contact with relatives:

- The nurse should identify him- or herself, the ward and the hospital clearly and slowly, confirm to whom he or she is speaking and the relationship with the patient.
- The nurse must explain clearly that the person has either been admitted to the accident and emergency department or a ward, or that the person's condition has unexpectedly deteriorated.
- The nurse must reassure the family that everything possible is being done; this may give relatives an insight into the seriousness of the patient's condition.

• If the nurse asks the family to come to the hospital he or she could suggest that they should be driven by someone if possible, thus suggesting that the situation is serious.

The nurse must be aware that the family may be angry if they arrive too late and she or he must always be truthful and say whether the patient was already dead when the phone call was made. If the family is not told the truth, then feelings of guilt of not being with the patient may ensue. If there is anger, the nurse must acknowledge it and be aware of their grief. Gently explain the reasons why you felt that this was the best way to break the sad news and apologize if the family feels that it was the wrong approach.

When people are distressed the nurse may find it difficult to know what to say, especially if he or she does not know the family. It is important to be gentle, warm and honest in approach. Any offer of help may be rejected, especially if relatives are unhappy about the care given to their loved one. If appropriate, touch may be appreciated by the grieving relative; however, the nurse must be aware of when to withdraw, but never be afraid to show that he or she cares because relatives gain comfort when nurses show emotion on the death of their loved one. Fraser and Atkins (1990) identified that some relatives have a vivid recollection of their experiences and the doctors and nurses to whom they spoke, whereas others remember nothing at all.

The hospital should accommodate the wishes that the relatives may have because it helps the grieving process. The relatives should be given refreshments in private. If they were not present at the death, they may wish to discuss the death with a nurse.

The nurse explains what will happen next: that the last offices will be carried out and the body transferred to the mortuary. The nurse also explains that the certificate stating the cause of death must be presented to the Registrar of Deaths, Births and Marriages in the area where the death occurred to obtain a death certificate, so that the undertaker can remove the body from the mortuary for burial or cremation. However, if the death does not occur in hospital and was expected, the patient's doctor will be contacted. The doctor will certify the cause of death and give the relatives a medical certificate stating the cause of death in a sealed envelope for the Registrar of Deaths, Births and Marriages, with a formal notice that states that the doctor has signed the medical certificate and tells the relatives how to register the death. As stated previously the death must be registered in the district where it occurred.

In the case of an unexpected death, if the district nurse finds the body, the patient's family doctor must be contacted. The police will then contact the dead person's nearest relatives if known and their minister of religion. If the cause of death appears not to have occurred from natural causes nothing should be touched.

If the death was known to be caused by natural illness but the doctors wish to know more about the cause of death, they may ask permission from the relatives to carry out a postmortem examination. The relatives may give their consent or withhold it. Reporting a death to the coroner occurs under the following circumstances:

- If the deceased person was not attended by a doctor during the last illness or within the last 14 days of life
- If the cause of death is uncertain or unknown
- If the death was sudden or occurred in suspicious circumstances
- If the death occurred following an accident or injury
- If the death occurred during surgery or recovery from an anaesthetic
- If the death occurred in police custody or in prison
- If the death occurred as a result of an industrial disease
- If the death occurred as a result of a notifiable disease.

The coroner is the only person in these circumstances who can certify the cause of death. The attending doctor will write on the formal notice that the death has been referred to the coroner. The coroner may require a postmortem examination of the body to ascertain the cause of death. The relatives are informed but their permission is not needed; however, they can choose for their own doctor to be present. If the postmortem examination shows that death was the result of natural causes the coroner may issue 'The Pink Form', which gives the cause of death for registration. A postmortem examination ordered by the coroner may or may not lead to an inquest; the purpose of the inquest is to ascertain the identity of the deceased in public and where, when and how the deceased died. The coroner is in control of the proceedings and there may be a jury if it is in the public interest to have one.

Last offices

An opportunity to view the body should be offered to the family either before laying the body flat or after the last offices have been performed. 'Last offices' is the last act that nurses are privileged to carry out for a patient for whom they have cared. The family must always be offered the opportunity to participate in this procedure, but must never be forced to do so; the nurse must be aware of both cultural and religious requirements. The nurse must have confirmed with the family what they want done at the time of the patient's death. In some cultures it is the members of the family or their religious group who perform the last offices. It must also be remembered that the way the body is handled forms an important part of how the bereaved view the hospital care and also helps them in their grieving process. Neuberger (1994) claims that it is essential that the correct procedures be followed during last offices, so that the wishes of the patient and the relatives are met, thus also ensuring holistic care. However, if they are disregarded we disregard both the patient's and the family's dignity (Speck 1988).

Most people have a spiritual aspect to their psyche. Some people call it their soul, others the inner energy that makes them whom they are.

Spirituality is frequently linked to religious beliefs. Firth (2001) claims that the lack of research into the spiritual and religious needs of ethnic minorities may be the result of the belief that religious and spiritual care are provided by the faith communities.

Equipment for performing the last offices

- A bowl, soap, two towels, two face cloths
- A razor, comb, nail scissors and nail file
- Equipment for cleaning dentures and oral toilet
- Notification of death labels and two identification bracelets
- A shroud or patient's nightdress or pyjamas or clothes requested by the patient or family, or those needed for religious or cultural observance
- A body bag may be required if there is the possibility of leakage of body fluids or an infectious disease
- Dressing pack with tape or bandages if there are any wounds
- Sellotape
- Valuables envelope, valuables book and property book
- Skip for dirty linen and plastic bag for waste
- Mortuary sheet.

All equipment must be taken to the bedside. The nurse should wear an apron and gloves. Patients in the beds nearby should be informed. All drainage tubes should be removed, unless otherwise stated, and covered with an occlusive dressing.

Wash the patient gently if permitted to do so by the family. A male patient may need to be shaved. The family may wish to assist in this procedure as a mark of respect for the loved one (respect and dignity must be afforded to the patient's relatives and the patient's body at all times). It must be remembered that nurses may not be permitted to carry out this procedure as identified earlier on religious and cultural grounds.

When turning the body over to wash the back, air that is trapped may be expelled. Some nurses find it easier to speak to the body as they did when the patient was alive.

The patient's mouth should be cleaned using a foam stick to remove any dry secretions or debris. If the patient has a wound, remove the soiled dressing and replace with a clean one. Dress the patient in a disposable shroud or his or her own clothes, depending on the policy of the hospital or relatives' requests.

Jewellery should be removed from the body unless otherwise stated by the family. This should be documented on a 'Notification of Death' form (or as per policy). The patient's valuables should be checked with another nurse, recorded and placed in a sealed envelope and stored according to hospital policy. If the family wish to view the body before it is removed from the ward, they should be given the opportunity to say their last farewells.

A patient's identification bracelet should be placed on the patient's wrist and ankle. A death notification label should be placed on the shroud. The body should be wrapped in a mortuary sheet, ensuring that the head and feet are covered and the legs secured in position by gently tying a tape around the two big toes. The sheet is then secured with Sellotape and the remaining death notification label is placed upside down on the sheet.

The portering staff should be notified to remove the body. However, a nurse must accompany them when they arrive to ensure that the body is removed gently and with respect.

Clear away soiled linen and waste in accordance with hospital policy. Remove gloves and apron. The patient's property should be sent to the appropriate administrative office. The bed should be washed thoroughly and disinfected in accordance with hospital policy before being remade. The nurse should also be aware of the needs of the other patients on the ward and be ready to answer their questions without breaching confidentiality.

Cultural and religious beliefs

Dickenson et al. (2000) claim that religion today is a philosophical attitude for many people, and not everyone apportions the same relevance to God and the afterlife as in previous generations. It is very important for the nurse to find out what the patient fears most, because the patient can communicate more fully with the nurse who empathizes with these fears.

Linton (1945) states that: 'the culture of a society is the way of life of its members; the collection of ideas and habits which they learn, share and transmit from generation to generation.' Our culture is learned from the place and group in which we grow up. It is made up of values, beliefs, attitudes and social awareness. It must be remembered that people brought up in the same area may have different cultural and religious beliefs. In many instances culture and religion are inseparable and the nurse must realize that people's beliefs may be complex.

Let us consider broadly some of the needs of certain religious groups, remembering that within these groups there are variations about what occurs at the time of death. The only way to be sure and not to offend is to ask (Table 15.1).

Bereavement

Bereavement is a normal process following the death of a loved one. Murray-Parkes' (1986) classic study of grief identifies four stages of bereavement: (1) alarm, (2) searching, (3) anger and guilt, and (4) depression/apathy/ gaining a new identity.

Alarm

The fight or flight response mirrors a stress reaction and lasts for between a few hours and 10 days. It displays itself through restlessness, panic, muscle tension, headaches, loss of appetite, insomnia and emptiness.

Table 15.1 Needs of certain religious groups

Religion	At time of death	After death occurs
Christianity	The patient may wish to recite prayers with the family. The priest or minister may be called to perform the blessing of the sick	Offices are performed according to hospital practice. A Christian may choose to be buried or cremated
Judaism	There is a wide variety of observances within the Jewish faith. The nurse must always respect the patient's and family's wishes. The patient may wish to recite prayers with the family	The body should be handled as little as possible. In some instances the family will carry out the last offices themselves. Jewish people are usually buried within 24 hours of dying
Islam	Prayers may be recited by the family as the patient faces Mecca	Non-Muslims should not touch the body. The last offices will be carried out by the family and Muslims are usually buried within 24 hours of dying
Sikhism	The patient and family may recite passages from the Holy Book	The family may wish to be involved with the nurses in carrying out the last offices. If the patient has taken the vow to abide by the five articles, this means they wear a short sword, a wrist band, cotton shorts, a wooden comb and never cut their hair, which in men is covered by a turban. The nurse should never remove any of these articles or cut the hair. Sikhs are always cremated as soon after death as possible
Hinduism	The Hindu priest may perform the holy rites and the patient may receive comfort from hymns and readings	The body should be touched only by Hindus. No jewellery or sacred threads should be removed from the body. All Hindus are cremated
Buddhism	Chanting by fellow Buddhists may help to relax the patient's state of mind which is very important	The last offices may be carried out according to hospital practice. Most Buddhists are cremated and their ashes are buried

From Green (1992).

Searching

This involves pining for the bereaved and pangs of yearning, the urge to search and find a reason for the death, and returning to the place where the death occurred.

Anger and guilt

These feelings are immense during the first month, together with intermittent periods of apathy and depression. There may be a tendency to blame others, frequently health professionals or God, for allowing it to happen and blaming the deceased for leaving them.

Depression/apathy/gaining a new identity

The bereaved person begins to feel the despair, empathy and pain of loss. There may be a loss of identity, e.g. if you lose a husband or wife whom you love, you lose a lover, friend, partner, confidant and in some instances the breadwinner.

Grief may be experienced in waves of extreme emotions but normal grief should be resolved over a period of time. Kubler-Ross (1969) claims that acceptance and integration into a new identity take five years. However, it must be remembered that grief is painful but normal and the person will find occasions such as birthdays and anniversaries sad and lonely times.

Coming to terms with the loss of a loved one is like having to come to terms with enforced change, with the loss of hopes, ambitions and dreams. If the bereaved person's grief is not resolved normally, they may have to be referred to a bereavement counsellor to help them reach the acceptance stage.

Although the stages described here demonstrate some understanding of grief, they are open to criticism in that people may not follow this or any pattern of bereavement. Some people may wish to maintain a connection with the deceased and not let them go completely (Klass et al.1996).

Russell (2002) claims that recent studies highlight people's individual experiences of grief that may be influenced by culture and social norms. Western societies expect the bereaved to resolve their grief in a short time span; however, for many people it is a long and painful journey.

Breaking bad news

Buckman (1984) said: 'by "bad news" I mean any information likely to alter dramatically a patient's view of his or her future.' Bad news being conveyed may not be about impending death but could be a diagnosis of diabetes, heart disease or HIV. The patient should be given the opportunity to ask questions, which should be answered sensitively, honestly and with empathy. The patient and family need to be reassured that help will be available if needed and that the nurse understands that they may not have taken all the implications in, and if they wish to make further appointments to ask more questions they must feel free to do so. Maguire and Faulkner (1988) claim that you cannot soften the impact of bad news because it remains bad news however it is broken, but it can be broken in a way that is supportive.

Kemp (1999) claims that patients and families frequently grieve for different losses, and that during the dying process they may progress at different speeds. Russell, in Hogston and Simpson (2002), claims that death may release many different emotions in people; some may be affected greatly and others less so. However, in some instances there may be relief as death means the end of suffering for their loved one.

Murray-Parkes (1986) describes grief as a psychosocial transition in which the bereaved person has to readjust his or her life without the deceased person, and has to realize that he or she has to adapt to a new and altered world. However, he claims that each person's experience of grief is unique. He also states that 'grief is essentially an emotion that draws us towards something or someone that is missing' (Murray-Parkes 2000).

Goodall et al. (1994) identify ways in which to help the bereaved:

- By being there
- By listening in a non-judgemental way
- By showing that you have some understanding of what they are going through
- By encouraging them to talk about the deceased
- By accepting silence
- By being aware of your own feelings about loss
- By offering reassurance that their grief is normal
- By not taking any anger personally
- By being aware that your feelings may reflect their own
- By resigning yourself to the fact that you cannot make them feel better.

Le Mone and Burke (1996) claim that the assessment of the bereaved person's social support systems is important because it helps in the normal outcome of their grief. However, in some instances loss of a loved one may lead to social isolation, with feelings of loneliness making the person withdraw from their usual social support systems; this results in the bereaved being in danger of prolonged abnormal grieving. The nurse must be aware of this and ascertain how often he or she meets friends and encourage him or her to continue doing so.

Conclusion

Caring for dying patients and supporting bereaved families is a demanding and sometimes stressful experience. If nurses are to offer the highest care they also need to be aware of their own needs. Loss, grief and bereavement will raise many professional and personal issues for all members of the multiprofessional health-care team. Each member of the team will need to support the others as well as the patient and the family.

It is important that a ward, community and hospice climate exists in which staff are seen to be sincere, sensitive and supporting because this will allow nurses to discuss their painful experience and use the support available without feeling a loss of professional control.

References

Adams, J. (1997) ABC of palliative care: The last 48 hours. British Medical Journal 315: 1600–1603.

Beauchamp, T.L. and Childress, J. (2001) Principles of Biomedical Ethics, 5th edn. Oxford: Oxford University Press.

Bradbury, M. (2000) The good death. In: Dickenson, D., Johnson, H. and Katz, J.S. (eds), Death, Dying and Bereavement. London: Sage, pp. 59–63.

Buckman, R. (1984) Breaking bad news: Why is it still so difficult? British Medical Journal 288: 197–199.

Buckman, R. (2000) Communication in patient care. In: Dickenson, D., Johnson, H. and Katz, J.S. (eds), Death, Dying and Bereavement. London: Sage, pp. 146–173.

Dickenson, D., Johnson, H. and Katz, J.S. (eds) (2000) Death, Dying and Bereavement. London: Sage.

Firth, S. (2001) Wider Horizons: Care of the dying in a multicultural society. London: The National Council for Hospice and Palliative Care Services.

Fraser, S. and Atkins, J. (1990) Survivors' recollections of helpful and unhelpful emergency nurse activities surrounding the sudden death of a loved one. Journal of Emergency Nursing 16(1): 13–16.

Freud, S. (1918) Reflections on War and Death. New York: Moffat Yard.

Goodall, A., Darge, T. and Bell, G. (1994) The Bereavement Training Manual. Bicester: Winslow.

Green, J. (1992) Death with dignity. Nursing Times 88(5): 36–37.

Henderson, V. (1996) The Nature of Nursing. New York: Macmillan.

Hockey, J. (1990) Experience of Death: An anthropological account. Edinburgh: Edinburgh University Press.

Hogston, R. and Simpson, P.M. (eds) (2002) Foundations of Nursing Practice: Making the difference, 2nd edn. Basingstoke: Palgrave Macmillan.

Jung, C.G. (1959) The Soul and Death. New York: McGraw-Hill.

Kemp, C. (1999) Terminal Illness: A guide to nursing care, 2nd edn. New York: Lippincott.

Klass, D., Silverman, P.R. and Nickman, S.L. (1996) Continuing Bonds: New understanding of grief. London: Taylor & Francis.

Kubler-Ross, E. (1969) On Death and Dying. New York: Macmillan.

Le Mone, P. and Burke, K.M. (1996) Medical/Surgical Nursing: Critical thinking on client care. Menlo Park, CA: Addison-Wesley.

Linton, R. (ed.) (1945) Present world conditions on cultural perspective. In: The Science of Man in World Crisis! New York: Columbia University Press.

MacDonald, B. and Rich, C. (1984) Look Me in the Eye: Old woman, ageing and ageism. London: The Woman's Press.

Maguire, P. and Faulkner, A. (1988) How to do it: communication with cancer patients. 2. Handling uncertainty, collusion and denial. British Medical Journal 297: 972–974.

Murray-Parkes, C. (1986) Bereavement. Harmondsworth: Pelican.

Murray-Parkes, C.M. (2000) Bereavement as a psychosocial transition, process of adaptation to change. In: Dickinson, D., Johnson, M. and Katz, J. (eds), Death, Dying and Bereavement. London: Sage, pp. 325–331.

Neuberger, J. (1994) Caring for Dying People of Different Faiths, 2nd edn. London: Mosby.

Russell, P. (2002) Social behaviour and professional interactions. In: Hogston, R. and Simpson, P.M. (eds), Foundations of Nursing Practice: Making the difference, 2nd edn. Basingstoke: Palgrave Macmillan, pp. 343–370.

Speck, P. (1988) Being There: Pastoral care in time of illness. London: SPCK.

Thayre, K. and Peate, I. (2003) Coping with expected and unexpected death. In: Hinchliff, S., Norman, S. and Schrober, J. (eds), Nursing Practice and Health Care, 4th edn. London: Arnold, pp. 291–314.

Thompson, N. (ed.) (2002) Loss and Grief: A guide for human services. Basingstoke: Palgrave.

Wilson, V. (2004) Supporting family carers in the community setting. Nursing Standard 18(29): 47–53.

Glossary of terms

Accessory organs: organs that contribute to digestion but are not part of the digestive tract.

Afebrile: absence of fever.

Allergen: an external substance that can stimulate an immunological response.

Alveolus: a terminal secretory portion of an alveolar duct (plural alveoli).

Amino acid: the building blocks of the body; an organic acid.

Angina: recurrent chest pain by physical or stressful events.

Antimicrobials: substances (usually medicines) given to destroy or prevent the growth of microbes.

Antipyretic: a drug used to control fever.

Anxiety: a mental state of uneasiness, apprehension or dread of perceived danger.

Anxiolytic: a drug used to treat anxiety.

Asepsis: absence of infection or infectious materials.

Attitude: a mental state that is made of many different beliefs, often involving positive or negative judgements about people.

Bacterium: the most common infection-causing micro-organism.

Basal laminar: the inner layer of the ciliary body.

Benign: the non-malignant characteristic of a neoplasm.

Body image: a mental picture an individual has of his or her own body and his or her feelings towards it.

Bradypnoea: respiratory rate less than 12 breaths/minute.

Bronchiole: a finer subdivision of the bronchi.

Bronchodilator: an agent that has the ability to cause an increase in the diameter of the bronchus.

Bronchospasm: contraction of the smooth muscle in the bronchi and bronchioles.

Buccal mucosa: mucosa adjacent to the cheek.

Cancer: a term used to describe any malignant disease.

Cardiac region: surrounds the cardiac orifice through which food enters the stomach.

Catabolism: break down in the body of complex chemical compounds.

Chemoreceptors: cells that respond to changes in a chemical environment.

Chromosomes: self-replicating structure of cells containing the cellular deoxyribonucleic acid (DNA).

Chyme: semi-solid substance containing partially digested food and gastric juices found in the stomach and small intestines.

Collagen: the major protein of the white fibres of connective tissue.

Colostomy: an opening of the colon on to the abdominal wall.

Corticosteroids: a group of drugs that are used to provide relief for inflamed areas of the body; they lessen swelling, redness, itching and allergic reactions.

Crepitations: crackling or a fine bubbling sound.

Cross-infection: infection caused when pathogens are transferred from one person to another.

Cutaneous: relating to the skin.

Cyanosis: a bluish or purplish discoloration (tinge) of the skin or mucous membranes.

Dementia: a progressive organic mental disorder characterized by personality changes, confusion, disorientation and a deterioration of intellect.

Dermatitis: inflammation of the skin.

Dignity: promoting self-respect and sense of worth.

Diurnal: repeating once every 24 hours.

Dyspnoea: shortness of breath, difficulty or distress in breathing.

Eczema: a general term for an inflammatory condition of the skin.

Electrolyte: chemical substances such as salts, acids and bases found in the blood and other body fluids.

Emphysema: an increase in the air spaces in the lung.

Emulsify: the dispersion of large fat molecules into smaller molecules in the presence of bile.

Endocrine: a ductless gland that secretes hormones into the bloodstream.

Endotracheal: within the trachea.

Enzyme: a substance that speeds chemical reaction.

Exocrine: a gland that secretes hormones into ducts which carry the secretions to other sites.

Febrile: relating to fever.

Gender: a social group's understanding of being a man or woman.

Haemoptysis: the coughing of blood from the lung or bronchial tree.

Heterosexuality: sexual attraction to or sexual relations with people of the opposite sex.

Homeostasis: a state of equilibrium of the internal and the external environment of the body.

Homosexuality: sexual attraction to or sexual relations with people of the same sex.

Hypothalamus: area of the brain that controls temperature, hunger and thirst.

Hypoxia: a decrease below the normal levels of oxygen in the tissues.

Hysterectomy: removal of the uterus.

Ileostomy: an opening of the ileum on to the abdominal wall.

Impotence: the inability to obtain/maintain an erection of the penis sufficient for sexual intercourse.

Integumentary system: the enveloping membrane of the body.

Ischaemia: lack of blood.

Libido: sexual drive.

Malignant: cancer that can invade the blood supply and the lymphatic system.

Mastectomy: excision of the breast.

Mastication: chewing process.

Merkel cells: cells of the epidermis believed to be involved with the sense of touch.

Metabolism: chemical and physical changes occurring within the tissues.

Micro-organism: a microscopic cell/organism.

Micturition: the act of passing urine.

Myocardial infarction: death of cardiac tissue caused by ischaemia.

Neoplasm: abnormal growth of tissue that may be benign or malignant.

NICE: acronym for National Institute for Clinical Excellence.

Nocturia: waking at night to pass urine.

Opiates/opioids: narcotic substances, e.g. morphine.

Organic disease: disease related to an organ.

Osmosis: diffusion of molecules via a semi-permeable membrane from a place of higher concentration to a place of lower concentration.

Osteoarthritis: degenerative changes within the joints.

Oximetry: the measurement, with an oximeter, of the amount of oxygen saturation of haemoglobin in the blood.

Palliative care: total care of a patient whose diagnostic condition is not curable.

Peristalsis: wave-like movements of the intestinal tract that help to move foodstuff down the intestine.

Pinna: part of the ear that projects outwards.

Postprandial: after a meal.

Prophylaxis: the prevention of disease.

Prostaglandins: hormone-like substances.

Pyloric region: funnel-shaped portion of the stomach where the pyloric sphincter is situated, which controls emptying of the stomach.

Pyrexia: core body temperature above 37.2°C.

Pyrogen: a fever-inducing agent that causes a rise in temperature.

Râles: small clicking, bubbling or rattling sounds in the lung.

Secondary sexual characteristics: physical attributes (other than the sexual organs) that distinguish males from females after puberty, e.g. facial hair in males and menstrual periods in females.

Self-awareness: being aware of one's own thoughts, feelings and actions.

Self-concept: the collection of ideas, feelings and beliefs that one has about one's self.

Self-esteem: the value one has for one's self.

Self-image: an individual's assessment of his or her own social worth.

Sensory receptors: specialized neurons that detect changes or respond to a stimulus.

Sepsis: the presence of pathogenic organisms or toxins in the blood or body tissues.

Serum: a clear watery fluid.

Sexual anomalies: deviation from the 'norm' – something that is unusual or irregular.

Sleep: an altered state of unconsciousness; the individual's perception of and reaction to the environment are decreased. This is a reversible state.

Solutes: the dissolved substance in a solution.

Somnambulance: sleep walking.

Steroids: a large family of chemical substances made up of many hormones.

Stoma: an artificial opening; Greek work meaning mouth.

Stratum basale: the deepest layer of the epidermis.

Stratum corneum: the outermost layer of the epidermis.

Stratum germinativum: provides the germinal cells necessary for the regeneration of the layers of the epidermis.

Stratum granulosum: the cells of the stratum granulosum provide lipids to help form a waterproof barrier.

Stratum lucidum: a layer found in the deepest layer of the stratum corneum – primarily found in the thick epidermis, e.g. palmar and plantar skin.

Stupor: a state of impaired consciousness.

Tachypnoea: an excessively rapid respiratory rate.

Tympanic membrane: the membrane that divides the middle ear from the external ear.

Ulcer: an erosion or loss of continuity of a mucous membrane, which may lead to suppuration.

Vestibule: enlarged area at the beginning of a canal.

Xerosis: pathological dryness of the mouth.

Xerostomia: dryness of the mouth – with various causes.

Normal values

The values given below are representative of the average reference range for adults in blood, cerebrospinal fluid and urine.

The ranges shown should be used only as a guide. Reference ranges between laboratories will vary; there are many reasons for this, e.g. the type of analytical equipment used and the temperature used, and you should always consult the ranges used in your own laboratory.

Blood (haematology)

Test	Reference range
Activated partial thromboplastin (APTT)	30–40 s
Erythrocyte sedimentation rate (ESR)	
Women	3–15 mm/h
Men	1–10 mm/h
Fibrinogen	1.5–4.0 g/l
Folate (serum)	4–18 µg/l
Haemoglobin (Hb)	
Women	11.5–16.5 g/dl
Men	13–18 g/dl
Hepatoglobins	0.3–2.0 g/l
Mean cell haemoglobin (MCH)	27–32 pg
Mean cell haemoglobin concentrate (MCHC)	30–35 g/dl
Mean cell volume (MCV)	78–95 fl
Packed cell volume (PCV or haematocrit)	
Women	0.35–0.47 (35–47%)
Men	0.4–0.54 (40–54%)
Platelets (thrombocytes)	$150–400 \times 10^9/l$
Prothrombin time	12–16 s
Red cells (erythrocytes)	
Women	$3.8–5.3 \times 10^{12}/l$
Men	$4.5–6.5 \times 10^{12}/l$
Reticulocytes	$25–85 \times 10^9/l$
White cells total (leukocytes)	$4.0–11.0 \times 109/l$

Blood venous (unless stated) plasma (biochemistry)

Test	Reference range
Alanine aminotransferase (ALT)	10–40 U/l
Albumin	36–47 g/l
Alkaline phosphate	40–125 U/l
Amylase	90–300 U/l
Aspartate aminotransferase (AST)	10–35 U/l
Bicarbonate (arterial)	22–28 mmol/l
Bilirubin (total)	2–17 µmol/l
Calcium	2.1–2.6 mmol/l
$Paco_2$ (arterial)	4.4–6.1 kPa
Chloride	95–105 mmol/l
Cholesterol (total)	< 5.2 mmol/l
HDL-cholesterol	
Women	0.6–1.9 mmol/l
Men	0.5–1.6 mmol/l
Copper	13–24 µmol/l
Cortisol (at 08:00 hours)	160–565 nmol/l
Creatine kinase (total)	
Women	30–150 U/l
Men	30–200 U/l
Creatinine	50–150 µmol/l
Globulins	24–37 g/l
Glucose (venous blood fasting)	3.6–5.8 mmol/l
γ-Glutamyltransferase (GY)	
Women	
Men	5–35 U/l
Glycosylated haemoglobin (HbA1c)	10–55 U/l
Hydrogen ion concentration (arterial)	4–6%
Iron	35–44 nmol/l
Women	14–32 µmol/l
Men	10–28 µmol/l
Iron-binding capacity – total (TIBC)	45–70 µmol/l
Lactate (arterial)	0.3–1.4 mmol/l
Lactate dehydrogenase (total)	230–460 U/l
Lead (whole blood)	< 1.7 µmol/l
Magnesium	0.7–1.0 mmol/l
Osmolality	275–290 mmol/kg
Pao_2 (arterial)	12–15 kPa
Oxygen saturation (arterial)	> 97%
pH	7.36–7.42
Phosphate (fasting)	0.8–1.4 mmol/l
Potassium (serum)	3.6–5.0 mmol/l
Protein (total)	60–80 g/l
Sodium	136–145 mmol/l
Transferrin	2–4 g/l
Triglycerides (fasting)	0.6–1.8 mmol/l
Urate	
Women	0.12–0.36 mmol/l
Men	0.12–0.42 mmol/l
Urea	2.5–6.5 mmol/l
Uric acid	
Women	0.09–0.36 mmol/l
Men	0.1–0.45 mmol/l
Vitamin A	0.7–3.5 µmol/l
Vitamin C	23–57 µmol/l
Zinc	11–22 µmol/l

Cerebrospinal fluid

Test	Reference range
Cells	0–5 mm^3
Chloride	120–170 mmol/l
Glucose	2.5–4.0 mmol/l
Pressure	50–180 mm/H$_2$O
Protein	100–400 mg/l

Urine

Test	Reference range
Albumin/creatinine ratio	< 3.5 mg albumin/mmol creatinine
Calcium (diet dependent)	< 12 mmol/24 h (normal diet)
Copper	0.26–0.6 µmol/24 h
Cortisol	9–50 µmol/24 h
Creatinine	9–17 mmol/24 h
5-Hydroxyindole-3-acetic acid (5HIAA)	10–45 µmol/24 h
Magnesium	3.3–5.0 mmol/24 h
Oxalate	
Women	40–320 mmol/24 h
Men	80–490 mmol/24 h
pH	4–8
Phosphate	15–50 mmol/24 h
Porphyrins (total)	90–370 mmol/24 h
Potassium[a]	25–100 mmol/24 h
Protein (total)	No more than 0.3 g/l
Sodium[a]	100–200 mmol/24 h
Urea	170–500 mmol/24 h

[a]Depends on intake.

Index